'HEAL THYSELF'

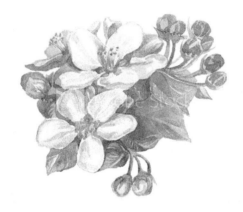

Dr. Alexander Haskell, ND

TABLE OF CONTENTS

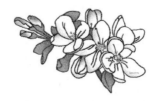

Introduction To Medicine

Let's start with a few guidelines or principles for those people interested in pursuing a medical approach which is not mainstream but rather 'alternative' or 'holistic.'

Please keep in mind that our present medical system, born in the antibiotic era, has existed for a relatively brief period of time and that what is now labeled as alternative has a rich history all the way back to Hippocrates.

People are waking up to the fact that modern medicine, when addressing chronic ailments, has its drawbacks.

Prescriptions do not 'cure' chronic ailments. They certainly offer relief, at least temporarily, but in the end, they do not in any way restore health.

Here are two typical scenarios people face when consulting their physician.

The 1st scenario ends with a person being told by their physician that all their lab results are normal, even though the person does not feel well. The doctor suggests that their condition must be due to stress, genetics, a psychological issue or that their symptoms are simply due to ageing.

The 2nd ends with a person being given a diagnosis and a prescription or referral.

1

Neither offers an explanation as to <u>why</u> or what the <u>causes</u> are for the person's condition.

People are realizing that they would prefer finding out why they are not well, to investigate the causes, and address them through more natural therapies and changes in eating habits and lifestyle.

People are becoming more open to alternatives because they don't want to take a prescription for the rest of their lives and because their doctor hasn't really been able to help.

Yet most people have no idea where to turn or how to find help from an alternative practitioner.

People are searching for two things; a cure for their symptoms without creating a drug dependency and answers to the question of why they don't feel well.

For a person to step outside our modern medical system and to search for an alternative takes courage.

From people's experiences and 'medical' indoctrination we've developed a medical mindset and have become accustomed to the traditional doctor's appointment.

- Tell the doctor their symptoms
- Have a physical exam and lab testing
- Receive a name (diagnosis) for their condition
- Receive a prescription or a referral

This approach doesn't place any demands upon the patient, meaning they don't have to take any personal responsibility for their condition or symptoms.

They just follow the doctor's orders.

Some people prefer this.

'Just give me a pill, doc.'

Yet this passive attitude of accepting the counsel of an authority, a lack of engagement and 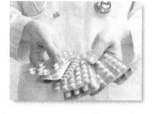 taking personal responsibility for one's recovery will, in the end, fail.

People with this same attitude or mindset may also expect a similar approach from an alternative practitioner, that a natural pill (supplement or herb) will bring them the relief they are seeking.

But 'fixing' chronic symptoms or a chronic illness is not so simple.

Why?

Because chronic illnesses result from an accumulation of causes or insults including;

- Stress
- Years of eating poorly
- Poor digestion
- The ingestion of pharmaceuticals and over-the-counter medications leading to gut issues and mitochondrial dysfunction
- Exposure to molds
- Heavy metals
- Our relentless exposure to thousands of chemicals in our water, food and environment
- Bacterial and viral infections in the past which never completely disappeared
- Compromised pathways of detoxification (liver, colon, kidneys and skin)
- Possibly an unsuspected dental issue
- Insomnia which doesn't allow the body to recover and

rejuvenate

These causes of illness will never be resolved by taking either a pharmaceutical or a 'natural' pill.

If a person simply seeks supplements as an alternative to a prescription this is, of course, their freedom of choice.

Yet I have witnessed those who have truly succeeded in recovering their health have done so because of their involvement.

Involvement means becoming educated about all the factors which either promote or sabotage our health.

Education must increase our awareness around toxins, chemicals and other causes of illness, and how to recognize and avoid them.

It means avoiding foods which are harmful while learning new habits of eating.

It means engaging in health promoting therapies.

It means recognizing and honoring their innate capacity to heal and to begin trusting and listening to their own instincts, intuition and common sense.

It means understanding that symptoms are the body's means of communication, and that we must learn its language and begin to investigate why we are experiencing symptoms.

Tipping the Scales

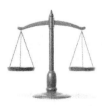

Here I use the symbol of the Libra Scale to explain the onset of symptoms and the development of a chronic illness.

When we are born the scale is tipped to one side, let's say all the way to the right.

This right side represents everything which promotes health including sunlight, fresh air, clean water, nutrient dense foods, a clean shelter, love, movement, creativity and a spiritual orientation to life.

The left side of the scale represents everything which is harmful and destructive to life.

These insults include pollution, synthetic chemicals, chronic anxiety and stress, pathogens, a sense of isolation and many others.

As these insults are slowly loaded onto the left side, the scale begins to tip towards the left.

This represents the onset of physical and mental symptoms, when the body and mind are trying to communicate to us that something is wrong.

The most important part to remember from the Libra Scale analogy is this.

When symptoms appear, we may THINK we know what caused them because the last 'thing' or insult placed on the left side caused the scale to slightly tip in that direction.

But it's important to understand that the scale didn't tip just because of this last 'thing' but because, over years and decades, many other insults had already been stacked on the left side.

It's the accumulation of many insults that tipped the scale and not just the one 'thing.'

People come in with what they believe to be the 'reason' why they became sick and they've seen many doctors without much relief.

Some examples I refer to which caused an obvious decline in their health are Lyme Disease, Epstein Barr Virus, mold exposure, heavy metal poisoning, exposure to a specific chemical, the replacement of mercury amalgam fillings, a parasite, a bad reaction to a drug, and many others.

But it was not until one more insult was placed on the left side that finally caused the scale to tip.

To some degree this may explain why many people with elevated EBV or Lyme Spirochetes feel perfectly well. They just don't have a lot of other insults piled on the left side.

To simplify this model, chronic illness results when we do not put enough beneficial things on the right side and are not conscious of the insults being loaded onto the left.

When we advance from symptoms to a full-blown chronic illness or disease, the scale has finally tipped all the way to the left.

As you can see from this model, you can place all the vitamin supplements in the world on the right side, but they will never be enough to tip the scale all the way back to health.

To recover our health, we must simultaneously remove insults from the left, avoid them as best we can and load more benefits onto the right.

Feeding the right side of the scale seems pretty obvious; organic nutrient dense foods, purified water, movement, fresh air, sunshine, a sense of purpose and belonging, specific herbs and supplements and many others.

When it comes to addressing the left side, this is bit more challenging.

Certainly the 1st step is to avoid what is harmful; pesticides, herbicides, chemicals, drugs, mold, common household cleaners, fluoride, heavy metals, artificial ingredients and sweeteners, pathogens and many others.

OK, so it's one thing to avoid these insults but it's another to remove them from the left side of the scale.

This is where various purification and specific intravenous therapies come in which will be covered soon.

Traditional vs. Alternative

As you can see there's a wide gap between the approach of our present medical system and the alternative.

Taking a prescription or over-the-counter medication will reduce symptoms yet these do nothing to shift the scale to the right.

In fact, any synthetic chemical will in the end make the situation worse because the drug and its residues would be placed on the left side.

The drug also silences your innate wisdom's attempt to communicate to you that something is wrong, that something is out of balance.

When a troubling symptom disappears because it is masked by a drug then you won't investigate its cause.

So, if you are considering the alternative path you need to understand the necessity of becoming involved.

I have been in practice as a Naturopathic Physician for 35 years and have seen over 4,000 new clients.

I have seen and heard just about everything.

Here is a typical theme.

They come in with a diagnosis like Lyme or cardiovascular disease or chronic fatigue or fibromyalgia or whatever the label may be.

But no matter what the condition, they all have very similar underlying 'issues' like blood sugar dysregulation, adrenal exhaustion, suboptimal hormones, a weak immune system, a history of eating poorly, drug use, poor gut ecology and digestive absorption issues.

Now if we venture even deeper into these causes, we find the body is burdened by toxins and chemical residues, low grade silent bacterial, viral and mold infections, severe nutrient deficiencies, compromised pathways of detoxification and others.

The person's current diagnostic label simply focuses on their most superficial health issue without considering causes and susceptibilities, and if therapies focus directly and solely on this diagnosis it will end in frustration since other underlying insults are not being addressed.

Yes, we must implement therapies which do address the uppermost issue yet must also cover the issues beneath the surface as well.

I want to reiterate this single point again because it is so very important.

You have received a diagnosis based on blood test results, a physical exam, and possibly a scan.

It is very easy to get stuck, thinking this is the 'thing' to treat and if this is 'treated' then your health will be restored.

It won't!

You may be relieved of symptoms to a certain degree, but you won't feel completely well.

Why?

Because all the other insults or issues that were there before (on the left side of the scale) are still there.

So yes, direct therapies to this uppermost issue BUT at the

same time help your body to excrete toxins and waste products stored in various tissues, become more aware of exposure to chemicals, and determine if there are lingering, low-grade, chronic infections.

In my experience with clients, those that stuck it out, who dove deep into the core of the multiple causes for their illness often expressed how their illness put them on a path that changed their life for the better.

They have a much deeper understanding of what is beneficial to them and what is not.

They trust their instincts much more than before.

They now take the time to engage in activities which are beneficial to their physical and mental health.

They are more in tune with the wisdom of the physician residing within them.

They have removed chemicals and toxins from their home, office, bathroom and kitchen.

They understand the importance of organic foods.

They are much less anxious when symptoms arise and use various natural therapies to correct them.

For them, recovering their health became a journey of self-awareness, self-empowerment and independence.

Not only did they increase their health but are now practicing preventative medicine, knowing that their quality of life is far better than before and that their longevity has been advanced.

This has been a brief introduction, an overview of how illness develops and how drugless therapies help to restore physical and mental health.

Basic Naturopathic Principles

Illness does not arrive like a thief in the night but gradually and silently seeps into our life.

There must be reasons for this.

There must be causes!

I believe that under utopian conditions (environmental, social, financial & political) we should be able to live out our lives in perfect health.

Yet this ideal is seldom the case and we naively call upon our highly advanced, technologically sophisticated system of medicine for the cure.

But the system does not take into consideration the multiple causes of chronic disease. This is in part due to the pharmaceutical industry's influence upon the education of physicians and this industry's lack of concern for addressing causes.

Why is it that so many known chemical carcinogens are dismissed by our FDA and EPA as being harmless though research has proven the opposite to be true?

How long will we continue to entrust our health to our government and for-profit corporations?

How has our society become so naïve about the long-term potential side effects of synthetic drugs?

We have strayed from the art of medicine which historically considered symptoms as the body's struggle to bring itself back into balance and regulation.

Of course, there are the compassionate, conscientious and well-intended physicians but they fall beneath the shadow of a multi-billion-dollar industry which does not promote health as much as it does shareholder profits.

But many people <u>are</u> seeking the light, realizing that drugs are not the answer.

Symptoms Are the Messenger

Let us first be clear about physical and mental symptoms, their origin and what they truly mean.

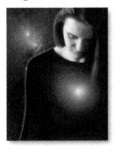

I strongly believe that everyone possesses the capacity to heal and I refer to this capacity as an innate wisdom which is superior in knowledge to the most enlightened physician.

I recall the subject of physiology in pre-med with the 1st chapter being devoted to homeostasis, the ability of the body (innate wisdom) to maintain the biochemical and hormonal balance of hundreds if not thousands of mechanisms within a healthy range.

I was extremely fortunate to have a professor who continued to remind us of this miraculous capacity, that the body possesses this incomprehensible ability to monitor, regulate

12

and correct any deviation from 'normal.'

Over the years I've come to understand more deeply how this wisdom has been actively and untiringly engaged in maintaining this balance ever since the moment of conception, day in and day out, until this present moment in time.

Describing it as miraculous is an understatement.

This means we each possess our own inner physician which has the ability to restore and maintain our health, while communicating to us through the language of physical and mental symptoms.

This communication is especially strong in children during an acute condition with symptoms of fever, sore throat, perspiration, fatigue or diarrhea.

Their inner physician is doing all it can to eradicate an invader while maintaining homeostasis.

In this example, we wouldn't want to negate or nullify these symptoms artificially but rather to support them.

My mother said that I could swim before I could walk but ear infections did occur occasionally. Warmed olive oil dripped into my ear was the common remedy.

I do recall one horrific ear infection around seven years of age and remember being escorted with my mother into the doctor's examination room.

After peering into my sore ear, he turned and faced a counter. Then turning around towards me he exposed a glass syringe with what appeared to be a 6-inch-long needle.

Horror struck, and my rebellious spirit rose from the depths of my being. Two nurses and the doctor could not hold me down for the injection of penicillin and eventually they gave up.

That night my fever rose again, and I broke into a heavy sweat, waking the next morning full of energy and a voracious appetite.

Of course, antibiotics may be needed if the child is unable to overcome the infection, yet both my mother and I learned two important lessons.

First is that the body has an incredible ability to fight and overcome infections and, second, that nothing could ever hold me back when I've made up my mind.

This same principle of listening to and respecting symptoms is also true for less acute issues such as mild aches and pains, dizziness, fatigue, headaches or an upset stomach after eating.

These symptoms are meant to communicate to us that something is not right, that we need to consider and investigate the reasons rather than turning to a drug or over the counter medication to reduce the symptoms.

I believe this is the most important mindset for anyone trying to recover their health, to understand that there are <u>always</u> reasons, <u>always</u> causes.

I do believe that health is the natural in-born state of a human being and that any deviation from this always has reasons.

Keeping this in mind, it must be the primary role of the individual and their physician to discover and uncover these reasons.

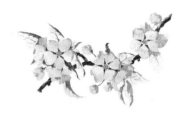

THE THREE PRIMARY CAUSES OF CHRONIC ILLNESS

Nutritional Deficiencies

So, here are some thoughts to consider around the causes of illness.

Over 2,000 years ago the Father of Medicine, Hippocrates, believed chronic ailments had two primary causes.

The 1st cause is nutritional deficiencies.

This makes common sense.

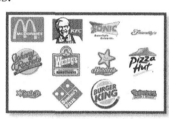

If our cells do not receive the nutrients they require to function optimally then naturally our physical and mental health will decline.

For many, this state of semi-starvation manifests in a wide variety of symptoms yet seldom do we or our physicians consider our symptoms being partly due to nutrient deficiencies.

Then there was Dr. Weston Price, DDS, who studied the effects of food upon health and disease.

He performed one of the most elegant nutritional research studies which supports the first cause of illness stated by Hippocrates, that of nutritional deficiencies.

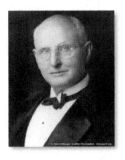 While practicing dentistry during the late 1800s and early 1900s Price was curious as to why children presented with far more dental issues than their parents.

His practice was during the time of advancing technologies in the processing and manufacturing of foods from companies like Kellogg's and Nabisco.

Price wondered if these dental changes might be due to the introduction and consumption of these less nutritious, industrialized foods.

So he decided to visit isolated regions of the world where people's nutrition was still restricted to locally grown foods.

Dr. Price and his wife traveled to the Swiss Alps, the coast of Scotland, Eskimo and Indian tribes in Canada, the aborigines of Australia, the Maoris of New Zealand, the Amazonian Indians and the tribesmen in Africa.

At that time these indigenous people lived in remote locations far from the influence of 'Western' foods and environmental toxins.

Price kept immaculate and journalistic style notes accompanied by photographs to illustrate his findings.

Price found that in each group every individual exhibited both dental and physical health.

Infirmities and disease were for the most part absent.

Tooth decay was extremely rare and dental crowding was nonexistent.

Over many decades Price returned to these communities to witness increased dental decay and a variety of chronic illnesses with the only variable being food stuffs imported by traders and missionaries.

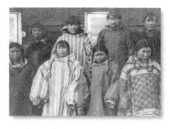

These new foods were primarily white sugar, refined grains, canned foods, pasteurized milk and 'devitalized' fats and oils.

These foods were not only less wholesome and nutrient deficient than local foods but also displaced the consumption of the foods normally eaten by these people.

If you have an interest in learning more about Dr. Price and to understand how our 'modern' foods are at the root of our epidemic in chronic illness, pick up a copy of *Nutrition & Physical Degeneration.*

Environmental Toxins

Of course, there are other insults which perpetuate chronic illnesses.

Hippocrates stated the 2nd cause of degenerative disease was toxins and many physicians over the centuries have also realized the negative impact environmental chemicals have upon health.

It seems obvious that when these foreign toxins enter our bodies in small yet persistent amounts, over time the body will express subtle symptoms which become progressively worse.

This is why a physician must investigate a client's living,

working and environmental surroundings, hobbies and gardening activities, food and water sources, mold exposure and even a chronological chemical exposure history.

Just because a person's symptoms developed recently, it's quite possible that a seed was planted decades before.

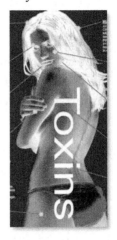

It is obviously futile to treat present symptoms without considering how and why, and the circumstances around which they developed.

So if our innate physician is communicating to us through physical and mental symptoms, how do we go about correcting the possible causes?

With toxins, the 1st step is to avoid or remove the cause or causes so that we are no longer being exposed.

The 2nd is to assist this innate wisdom to excrete them.

How to do this will be discussed later.

But there are other causes in addition to nutritional deficiencies and environmental toxins which other clinicians since Hippocrates have recognized as causative.

Pathogens

Louis Pasteur ushered in the germ theory, that micro-organisms were the cause of acute and chronic illness.

This is true but another 19th century French scientist, Claude Bernard, proposed that it was not just the pathogen but the person's susceptibility to the pathogen which led to illness.

This susceptibility, for why the person's own immune system

could not combat the infection, has to do in part with the two other causes of illness, nutritional deficiencies and the body's total burden of toxins.

Pathogens are then the third primary cause of illness but in most cases, these pathogens are silent, meaning they don't produce acute symptoms such as a fever but rather a host of chronic symptoms.

They are silent, low-grade and chronic, and normally don't show up on blood tests.

Before moving on to the next section I will summarize.

Our medical system has made many incredible advances and is certainly necessary at times, yet it is floundering when it comes to chronic disease and 'true' healing.

It creates dependency, seldom asks the patient to take responsibility for their condition, is dogmatic in its opposition to alternative medicine, places a huge financial strain on patients and our nation, negates or neglects the miraculous inner healing capacity of the person and does not address the causes for why a person has become ill.

Each person must exercise their common sense and to seek ways of health, ways which will do no harm, and which support their innate physician.

The process of healing and regaining one's full vitality takes time.

Patience, persistence and the practice of a new lifestyle are essential.

For many, illness can become a door through which they discover a calling and an opportunity to see life differently, to become educated and empowered, and to pursue a life that resonates more deeply with their heart and soul.

Therefore, do not fear leaving behind that which is not congruent with your ideals.

Stop struggling and begin to develop faith in your innate ability to heal.

Leave the past behind and find some solace in the here and now.

Surrender to your inner wisdom, for you are never alone.

Listen and trust this wisdom within whose whisperings are your instincts, your common sense and your intuition.

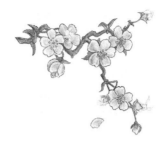

NATURE CURE

An ancient principle of medicine is that all true healing comes from nature and that nature provides all the elements the human body requires for health and healing.

Nature provides these elements in the air we breathe, the food and herbs we ingest, the water we drink and the sun we are exposed to, which is vital for every form of life.

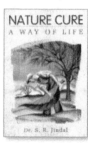

Nature is what we as physicians have called upon for centuries. Yet I wish to add an additional perspective.

Yes, nature provides the elements of healing, yet it is the Nature within you, this miraculous wisdom within, which uses and responds to these elements from nature.

The essence of Nature Cure revolves around the body's innate capacity to heal and your role is to assist it by providing what it requires to recover and to preserve your health.

This means becoming more in tune with this wisdom, to listen to its whisperings, to provide what it requires and to avoid what is harmful.

21

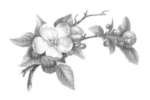

THE INNATE WISDOM
WITHIN YOU

The Mystery Within

I know this topic has been briefly covered already but I believe
it bears repeating.

One of the most influential teachers during my medical
education was Dr. Coppinger.

Sitting in an amphitheater classroom, his podium became a
theatrical stage as he portrayed the various biological and
biochemical characters in human physiology.

He would act out the intelligent
response of a white blood cell as
it detected and engulfed a
pathogen, or the dysfunction of
a nerve cell caused by the
paralyzing effects of a pesticide.

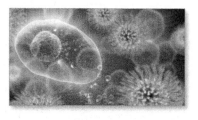

His enthusiasm and devotion to education brought life to the
science of physiology.

One subject he repeatedly wove into almost every lecture was
'homeostasis' or the body's innate ability to maintain a balance

in the body's biochemistry.

He was fascinated by this miraculous capacity. He helped us to realize that this innate wisdom is not located in any tissue or organ but permeates throughout our entire body.

Suddenly there was this new unseen, mysterious element which could not be explained or dissected.

We could only be a witness to its effects upon the body and mind.

It is a miraculous and unfathomable wisdom.

It is not of this physical world yet is fully integrated within every cell and tissue of your being.

This perspective is seldom considered by medical science even though it resides within each of us.

I hope this insight, this recognition of an innate invisible power being the source of healing will drive deep into your soul and bring with it a new sense of hope.

Life Force

From the moment of your conception this mysterious power ignited the flame of your earthly existence and you, as a single

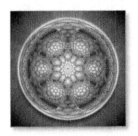

cell, began to split and multiply into a myriad of intricate biological and anatomical systems.

Hundreds, then thousands, then millions and trillions of cells evolved taking on their specific function within the hormonal, neurological and skeletal systems, all orchestrated by this mysterious power which has been functioning within you every second of the day and night.

Its intelligence knew exactly how to split one cell into trillions, so without a doubt it possesses the wisdom to recover your health and to maintain your well-being.

It is your true physician.

To refer to this innate intelligence as a miracle is an understatement, for its wisdom can never be truly understood by the finite mind of man.

And what is its essential purpose?

It is to serve you by maintaining your health and to help you live your life with more purpose and passion.

But to serve you it must communicate to you what is beneficial and what is harmful, and you must learn how to listen.

Its language is not through your mother tongue but rather through physical symptoms, instincts and intuitions.

It also guides you through the whisperings of your conscience.

Signs & Symptoms

Floating on the surface of our awareness are physical sensations and emotions. They can be pleasurable or unpleasant.

When we feel healthy, we don't experience physical or mental symptoms because our cells, tissues and glands are functioning well.

When our health gradually slips away, we then begin to experience symptoms.

We know the feelings or the bodily sensations of health but now we feel something is off. Maybe its fatigue or minor aches and pains, physical weakness or our concentration is not what it used to be.

The unpleasant physical ones are referred to as symptoms such as joint pains, headaches, a sense of fatigue, light headedness, nausea and others.

There is also a general sense that we just plain don't feel well and is challenging to describe.

When we see a physician, he or she is making observations and listing the patient's complaints.

The physician's observations are called signs and the patient's complaints are recorded as symptoms.

Signs are what the doctor observes.

Symptoms are what the patient complains of.

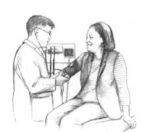 During a typical visit the physician may listen to the lungs, check blood pressure and pulse, examine the eyes and ears and palpate the abdomen.

The physician is searching for signs.

Then a routine blood test is ordered for blood sugar, liver and kidney function, red and white blood cells and others.

The gathering of all this information is with the hope of formulating a diagnosis.

Yet even with a diagnosis we should still pause to consider the causes of why we don't feel well.

My Doctor Says I'm Normal But I Feel Like...

In the first stage of dysfunction, when this innate wisdom is struggling to maintain homeostasis, lab results will seldom identify any abnormality and the doctor's physical exam may reveal nothing as well.

We know we don't feel well even though the doctor cannot discover anything abnormal.

This 1ˢᵗ stage of dysfunction can last a very long time.

The 2ⁿᵈ stage, usually years later, may present with more severity showing abnormal lab results and more obvious symptoms and signs.

This 2ⁿᵈ stage will often result in a diagnosis and prescription.

If symptoms are more on the mental-emotional plane, such as depression, with no abnormal lab results then you'll likely be referred to a psychiatrist.

The point here is that, during the 1ˢᵗ stage, labs may indicate tendencies. Results may fall within the lab's reference range yet are likely teetering away from optimal.

Probably half the people I've seen come in with this scenario.

'I feel sick, but my doctor tells me everything (lab tests) is normal.'

Remember, there are always reasons or causes for why we don't feel well and often the typical lab tests may only point towards tendencies.

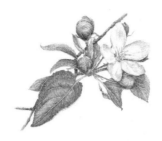

Second Model Explaining Symptoms & Chronic Illness

Here is another symbol or model which helps us to understand how we progress from health to illness.

This simple example was presented in our 2nd year of naturopathic medical school and has greatly influenced my approach with clients over the last 30 years.

Imagine an empty bowl. It represents the body's capacity to deal with our exposure and accumulation of toxins and applies to the 2nd and 3rd causes of illness.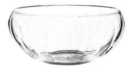

I include the 3rd cause because pathogens, i.e. bacteria, mold and parasites, excrete their waste products, called biotoxins, into our body leading to symptoms.

At birth the bowl is empty yet over time, as we are exposed to environmental toxins, chemicals and biotoxins, our bowl slowly fills.

Even during this filling period, we still feel fine, until the day our bowl becomes completely full and starts to spill over the edge.

This analogy of spilling over represents physical and mental symptoms, when the total body burden of toxins is greater than the body's capacity to handle and excrete them.

These symptoms tell us that something is wrong.

This is the stage when people visit their physician to be told that nothing appears wrong on lab tests, with people often resorting to over the counter medications to find relief.

This is why we may feel well up to a certain age, and then begin to experience symptoms and a gradual decline in our health.

This is why, unless we address this accumulation of toxins, we shall never regain our health through drugs and even natural remedies unless they address purification or the emptying of the bowl.

This transition from health to symptoms is often subtle and can be triggered by what seems to be a slight insult, yet it is the accumulation of toxins over years and decades which is the underlying cause for this decline.

So, using this model there are two actions to take.

Stop Filling the Bowl

The 1st is obvious, stop filling the bowl. Stop exposing ourselves to harmful influences.

Anything that comes in contact with our skin is absorbed into the body.

What we inhale enters our blood stream.

What we ingest enters both our blood stream and lymph system.

This reduction of exposure should be the basis of preventative medicine.

Empty the Bowl

The 2nd is to empty the bowl. If we can drain the bowl then we can advance towards our original state of health and vitality.

Some of you may remember what it felt like to have abundant energy, to run and play freely and to seldom feel exhausted.

I believe this abundant energy is still present and lies deep within you.

This energy will never be released by a pill or supplement.

Your symptoms will never truly recede and your vitality will never resurface until you empty your bowl of toxic, poisonous residues and biotoxins.

There are several means of emptying the bowl which will be covered in just a moment.

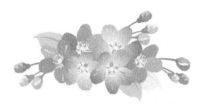

DEEP INTO THE CORE OF
CHRONIC ILLNESS

Every condition, and I mean it when I say EVERY condition has symptoms which are specific or localized, like headaches, and some symptoms which are general or systemic, such as fatigue and depression.

No matter what the symptoms might be, the issue comes down to cellular dysfunction, meaning that the origin of both localized and systemic symptoms relates to cells, which make up tissues and glands.

I ask, 'Where else but in our cells does illness reside?'

One approach, and maybe the most important one, is to improve the health and function of our cells, since this is what we are made up of, over 40 trillion of them.

So let's talk about a cell, and what causes a decline in its function leading to symptoms, and how to improve its health and activity.

Besides the nucleus of the cell, which contains our genetic material, what part of the cell provides the energy or the powering of the cell to express its function, whether it's a brain, liver, heart or thyroid cell?

33

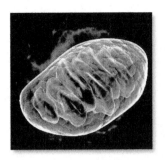 It is our mitochondria.

Mitochondria have several functions but, in this case, we will focus on their production of energy or ATP.

Almost every cell in the body has hundreds of these mitochondria, sometimes even thousands in cells which have a high metabolic rate, i.e. brain, liver and heart.

There are several causes or reasons for why our mitochondria can decline in their production of energy, which brings us back to the three primary causes of chronic conditions; nutritional deficiencies, environmental toxins and infections.

If our mitochondrial do not receive the nutrients they require then naturally their function will decline and symptoms will appear because of lowered energy production.

When we are exposed to various pollutants and chemicals, some of their residues are sequestered or compartmentalized inside our cells, and this causes a decline in mitochondrial function, often referred to as mitochondrial dysfunction.

Pathogens such as bacteria, mold and parasites secrete their metabolic waste, referred to as biotoxins. These find their way into our cells with the same effect as chemicals have upon our cells.

So the challenge then is to figure out a way to get these toxic residues out of our cells to improve their function and to restore our health at the cellular level.

To excrete toxic residues from within our cells requires an active transport, meaning it takes cellular energy, specifically ATP produced by our mitochondria, to clean up our cells.

So everyone with a chronic health issue is in a tight spot.

Toxic residues are inside our cells, which have caused mitochondrial dysfunction and lowered energy production, yet it takes energy to excrete them.

What to do?

Somehow we have to increase mitochondrial function.

So we are back to nutrition, to provide all the nutrients our mitochondria require to function optimally.

But the issue for many people with a chronic condition is that they don't have much of an appetite, and very often have digestive issues, of not breaking food down completely, and poor assimilation of nutrients from the gut into the body.

Taking a digestive enzyme which mimics the primary enzyme our stomach cells secrete, which is hydrochloric acid, can help.

Of course, you have to make some, likely many, dietary changes and consume nutrient dense foods.

To understand more about nutrition and the importance of feeding our mitochondria, watch a Ted Talk by Dr. Terry Wahls, MD, who recovered from MS primarily through nutrition.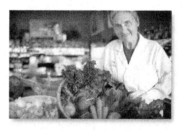

Assimilation issues are frequent and often come down to SIBO (Small Intestinal Bacterial Overgrowth), Candida and parasites.

Supplements are another important way to feed our mitochondria in order to increase the production of energy and aid in the detoxification of our cells.

We like one called Mitocore which is formulated with almost all the nutrients our tiny mitochondria need to function optimally.

The only nutrient missing in this supplement is Coenzyme Q10, taking 1-2mg per pound body weight.

You also might look into PQQ to improve not only the function of our mitochondria but to increase their number.

So this covers the feeding of your mitochondria.

Next, we'll cover ways to accelerate their function, all with the objective of getting toxins out of our cells.

Requirements for Cellular Function

Besides nutrients, our cells require two things to function.

The first is oxygen. No O2...we die.

The second is glucose. No glucose...coma.

Besides glucose, there are other fuels our cells can use, and one of them is like a high-octane fuel.

First, a little physiology.

Most of the food we consume is converted into glucose. This includes starches or carbohydrates, proteins, fats and fruit.

Carbs convert pretty rapidly while proteins and fats take longer.

After a meal, glucose in the blood increases.

Along the way, this glucose slowly leaves the blood and enters our cells to fuel the production of energy or ATP.

At this point the glucose in the blood is declining.

At some point our glucose declines to where it was before we ate, and it may continue to decline towards low blood sugar or hypoglycemia.

If there's not enough glucose in our blood, often the function of our cells declines and we experience symptoms; mental fog, dizziness, irritability and fatigue.

'Feed me!'

Usually we don't get to this point because people don't like to experience low blood sugar, so we snack between meals and listening for the early signs and symptoms, we eat.

This is typically our steady state from day to day, month to month, year to year, to continue eating three meals a day plus snacks.

It didn't always used to be this way when we look back through the centuries, when food might have been more sparse during certain seasons.

So what happens when the alarm, 'Feed Me,' goes off, and we don't eat?

The body's initial response to falling blood sugar is to click an alarm button, signaling the adrenal glands to secrete the hormone cortisol.

Cortisol is a steroid hormone made from cholesterol. I won't go into all the health issues when cholesterol is too low and the multiple side-effects of lipid lowering drugs.

Cortisol stimulates glycogenolysis, the breakdown of glycogen stored in various organs and tissues, which brings our blood glucose back to where it should be and brings us out of hypoglycemia.

Cortisol also has a lipolytic effect, the breakdown of fat inside fat cells to form free fatty acids and glycerol, which are transported to our cells calling out for glucose.

These fatty acids are then activated and transported into our mitochondria.

From here they are broken down and processed in the citric acid cycle, with the end result of increasing ATP production, even more so than what happens with glucose.

Both the above, the breakdown of glycogen and the release of free fatty acids from fat cells have other benefits as well as increasing ATP production.

Besides all our cells, fat cells are the primary storage sites used by the body to sequester toxins.

So the release of cortisol due to declining blood sugar is one method of detoxifying toxic residues from fat cells.

But remember, we are talking about recovering our overall health by increasing cellular mitochondrial function, which will detoxify all our cells by increasing ATP production.

To encourage this production, to actively transport toxins out of our cells, there are a few options.

The first is to fast intermittently, meaning to not eat for a short period of time, once in a while.

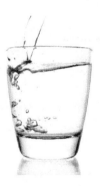

After finishing dinner, say around 7pm, you would not eat again until noon the next day, and consuming only water, not juices, because these would increase glucose.

Extended fasts would last from one day (24 hours) to longer periods, up to three day.

Longer than this might require some supervision.

Either way, whether it's intermittent fasting or the extended water fast, you may experience symptoms such as headaches, joint pains, nausea and fatigue as your cells are releasing toxins which have been stored up for years.

These symptoms are a good thing.

What…???

Yes, these are typical symptoms of detoxification, of emptying the bowl, of getting toxins off the left side of the Libra scale.

The only concern with this practical and effective approach of detoxification at the cellular level is, what happens to these toxins once they've exited our cells.

First, they enter the fluid outside our cells, the lymph, which is another storage site for toxins, and if a person leads a sedentary lifestyle, very likely their lymph is like a swamp, and these additional toxins will cause the person to feel even worse.

The lymph needs to move, and physical movement is important.

Hot and cold showers and alternating between and hot sauna and a cold shower will help with lymph movement.

So what happens to these toxins in the lymph?

Lymph drains through two channels or ducts into the blood stream and are carried through the blood to the kidneys and liver for excretion.

If you have kidney issues, beware. This approach takes some supervision.

There are herbal and homeopathic remedies to support and help kidney drainage.

The liver in most people has been working overtime and needs support.

From the liver, metabolized toxins enter the gall bladder. Again, another swamp and like the trash can of the body.

For both the gall bladder and liver, I recommend a product from Seeking Health, their gall bladder powder, taking 1-2 scoops once or twice daily in water on an empty stomach.

Once the toxic residues have left the liver and gall bladder, they travel to the small intestines, and must make their way through approximately 25 feet of intestines.

Reabsorption and recycling of these toxins becomes an issue.

To prevent this, a binder supplement will help prevent this recycling.

Binders can be clay, charcoal and many others.

Usually it's 2-4 capsules taken away from food on an empty stomach.

Of course, it's only common sense to avoid toxins in the fluids we drink, the foods we consume, the air we breathe and what we put on our skin.

We must increase our awareness, and not trust large corporations and agribusiness to have our interests at heart. It's about profits and shareholder, not the consumers.

There are other chapters which discuss more about the importance of detoxification.

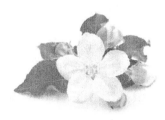

AN OVERVIEW OF OUR APPROACH TO CHRONIC HEALTH ISSUES

Now that we've covered some of the principles of wellness and the many causes of chronic illness, let's step back for a moment and look at some practical steps towards recovery.

Imagine a very ill woman whose condition is due to all the causes we've covered.

To understand how to help her, you must first know a little anatomy and physiology.

In the body there are three compartments of fluid; inside our cells, our lymph and our blood vessels.

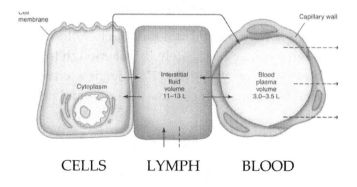

CELLS   LYMPH   BLOOD

Lymph fluid bathes every cell and has various key features;

- It's like a stream that flows through us.
- It carries nutrients absorbed from the intestines to our cells.
- Hormones leaving the blood travel through the lymph to cells.
- Lymph is another storage site for toxins exiting the blood.
- Waste released from our cells enters the surrounding lymph fluid.
- Lymph fluid drains into the blood stream where waste and toxins are then filtered and removed by the liver and kidneys.

So, this woman has the following issues which are causing her symptoms.

- All her cells are undernourished and are therefore under functioning. This can be due to a poor diet and/or poor digestion and/or poor assimilation of nutrients from the gut into the body.
- All her cells have accumulated toxic residues from her environment and her use of drugs.
- She has some bacterial and mold in her blood, not enough to make her acutely ill but enough to cause some degree of symptoms. Pathogens excrete their waste (biotoxins) which have also accumulated inside her cells.
- Because of the above, her mitochondrial are not functioning optimally and are therefore causing some

of her symptoms.

- This mitochondrial dysfunction has compromised her ability to excrete toxins from within her cells.

- Her immune system is under functioning. One important function of her white blood cells is to capture (phagocytize) impurities and dead pathogens in the blood.

- Her pathways of detoxification (liver, kidneys, intestines and skin) are compromised and unable to efficiently clear toxins.

- Her lymph system, which helps to carry away toxins from tissues, is clogged and is more like a swamp than a stream.

When toxins in the blood are filtered by the liver, they pass into the intestines to be excreted with the feces. These metabolized toxins have a negative impact upon digestion and assimilation of nutrients, and some toxins are likely to be reabsorbed back into the body since she has some degree of constipation.

Even if her cells could excrete toxins from within, with her lymph being stagnant with high concentrations of toxins, her cellular detoxification is greatly compromised.

So, what are the steps we can take towards helping her to recover her health?

We have several goals;

- Improve mitochondrial function

- Get toxins out of cells

- Reduce pathogens in the blood

- Improve lymph flow

- Increase the intake of nutrient dense foods

- Improve digestion and assimilation

- Optimize the pathways of detoxification

  o Liver; IVs, Supplements & Herbs

  o Kidneys; Supplements & Herbs

  o Intestines; Diet, Probiotics, Colon Hydrotherapy and others

  o Skin; Saunas

Yet, in what order do we approach all the above?

If we focus on restoring mitochondrial function and her cells begin excreting stored toxins into her stagnant lymph, she will feel worse, because she is unable to get them out of her body.

So this is would not be the initial focus of therapy.

We could begin with therapies to reduce the population of pathogens in her blood which would reduce the level of circulating biotoxins. This would help to improve immune function.

This is good.

We should improve lymph flow and turn her swamp into a stream. Lymphatic drainage, the Bemer, lymphatic hydrotherapy and the Photon Sound Beam unit will accomplish this.

But when lymph flow increases, many toxins will be dumped into the blood.

Therefore, we must improve liver and kidney function first in order to handle the additional toxins coming into the blood when lymph flow is increased.

Toxins filtered from the blood by the liver flow into the

intestines and travel through the entire intestinal tract to exit with the feces.

With this woman having constipation we must first get her bowels to work more efficiently otherwise the toxins filtered by the liver will be absorbed back into her body.

One therapy to help the intestines to rapidly eliminate these toxins is through colon hydrotherapy along with specific supplements like vitamin C and magnesium.

Another route of purification is through the skin.

The benefits of a dry heat or ozone steam sauna are immediate because perspiration carries toxins which have been stored in the subdermal fat layer, just under the skin.

So, here is a list of the therapies we offer which will be covered in more detail in upcoming chapters. Some are to improve nutritional status while others are for eliminating toxins, infections and drug residues.

- IVs to reduce pathogens
    - Zotzmann 10-Pass Ozone Therapy
    - UBI (Ultraviolet Blood Photonic Therapy)
    - High Dose Vitamin C
- IVs to restore optimal nutrient status and mitochondrial function
    - Vitamins, Minerals and Trace Minerals
    - BiOcean from France
    - Meyers Push of Nutrients
    - Phosphatidyl Choline for Cellular Membrane Repair
- IVs to Improve Detoxification through the Liver

- Alpha Lipoid Acid
- Glutathione
- IVs for Heavy Metal Detox
  - Calcium EDTA
  - Disodium EDTA
  - DMPS
- IVs for Drug & Chemical Cellular Drainage
  - NAD (Nicotinamide Adenine Dinucleotide)
- Lymphatic Drainage
  - Lymphatic Drainage Massage
  - Lymphatic Hydrotherapy
  - Photon Sound Beam
  - The Bemer for Clearing Lymph and Matrix
- Colon Hydrotherapy
- Saunas (Our Sauna Detox Program)
  - Dry Heat Walk-in Sauna with Cold Shower
  - Ozone Steam Capsule with Cold Shower

Details about all these therapies will be covered in the next few chapters.

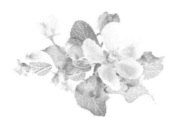

Intravenous Therapies
for Recovery

In this section we'll cover all our IV therapies which address nutritional deficiencies, pathogens and toxins.

Some IVs overlap when addressing these causes.

As an example, vitamin C is a nutrient and antioxidant, yet at higher concentrations it acts as an oxidant to improve mitochondrial function, reducing pathogens and the excretion of toxins.

Oxidative Type IVs for Pathogens

To discover if a person has issues with blood pathogens, we use both standard lab testing and the viewing of a tiny drop of a client's blood, sandwiched between two pieces of glass (a microscope slide and a cover slip), under a dark-field microscope.

To reduce bacteria including spirochetes, viruses and mold we provide the following IV therapies.

Zotzmann 10-Pass Hyperbaric Ozone

With ozone we are trying to mimic what our own immune system does.

Our white blood cells produce hydrogen peroxide which is H_2O_2.

This molecule breaks down into H_2O (water) and a singlet oxygen (O-) which kills or oxidizes pathogens.

Ozone, which is O_3, breaks down into O_2 and the same singlet oxygen.

Therefore, ozone has many health benefits including the reduction of bacteria, viruses and molds, increased oxygen carrying capacity of red blood cells and improved function of mitochondria.

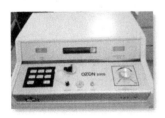

The German made Zotzmann machine allows us to mix ozone with nearly half the body's blood by treating 2,000cc or 2 liters at a single sitting.

This is usually about a two-hour treatment.

After almost two years of experimenting and checking results using the dark-field microscope before and then after the Zotzmann treatments, we have found the best results occur using intravenous vitamin C IV anywhere between 6 to 16 hours after a Zotzmann treatment.

I believe the Zotzmann has ushered in a new frontier of medicine especially when considering the increasing incidence of antibiotic resistant infections.

The Unit:

- The Zotzmann uses pure oxygen from an adjacent tank

to make ozone.

- The dial on the right side of the unit can be rotated to control the concentration of ozone.

- One end of a clear sterile IV line is connected to the Zotzmann unit with the other end inserted into a sterile glass, 200cc vacutainer.

- Through this line we control the pressure inside this vacutainer as well as the delivery of ozone into the vacutainer at the appropriate time.

- One end of another sterile IV line is inserted into the client's vein with the other end being inserted into the vacutainer.

- Through the Zotzmann we create a slight vacuum inside the vacutainer so that blood will flow rapidly from the vein into the vacutainer.

- When the blood in the vacutainer reaches 200cc we then press a button on the Zotzmann to deliver approximately 200cc of ozone under high pressure.

- The 200cc of ozone is mixed with the 200cc of blood inside the vacutainer to kill pathogens.

- Then another button on the Zotzmann is pressed, creating pressure inside the vacutainer to facilitate a rapid return of blood to the vein.

This 200cc of ozonated blood is considered a single pass and the typical treatment repeats this process nine more times, a total of 10 passes, thus the treatment of 2,000cc of blood.

Then between 6 to 16 hours after the Zotzmann we normally recommend an IV of vitamin C.

You can learn more about this therapy on our website at ClearHealthCenters.com.

UBI or Bio-Photonic Therapy

This ultraviolet blood therapy has been in use by physicians for over 70 years.

It is extremely safe and may be the best therapy for blood born pathogenic infections and immune system disorders such as Multiple Sclerosis, Lupus Erythematosus, Rheumatoid Arthritis and many others.

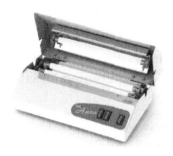

In the US we have about 250 practitioners using UV in their clinics.

There have been over a million treatments given and not a single adverse reaction recorded.

Some proven benefits of this therapy are the following:

- Kills bacteria, viruses and molds in the blood

- Supercharges the immune system

- Improves microcirculation

- Oxygenates tissues

- Reduces inflammation

- Stimulates red blood cell production

- Increases the flexibility of red blood cells and therefore better oxygen delivery to tissues

- Cardiovascular benefits due to increased circulation and oxygenation of muscles

Most clinicians using UBI will typically treat about 60cc of blood at a sitting.

We have greatly modified this by using the UBI unit pictured above in conjunction with the Zotzmann.

We use the same setup mentioned above, and when the ozonated blood is returning to the vein, it passes through a special clear glass line secured in the UBI unit.

So, to clarify, 200cc of ozonated blood travels from the vacutainer through the UV unit only when it is flowing toward the vein, not when it is coming from the vein.

This is done twice, allowing the treatment of approximately 400cc of blood.

We have found this method far superior to treating just 60cc of blood.

At no time is the catheter or needle removed from the client's vein, so every step remains sterile.

Here is a partial list of some conditions that have responded well to this UV therapy.

- Lymphoma
- HIV
- Hepatitis
- Herpes zoster and simplex
- Shingles
- Mononucleosis
- Viral pneumonia
- Polio
- Wound infections
- Fibromyalgia
- Lupus
- Rheumatoid arthritis

- Psoriasis
- MS
- Fungal and yeast infections
- Cirrhosis of the liver
- Chronic fatigue
- Septicemia infections
- Severe acne
- Scleroderma
- Asthma
- Sinus infections
- Bronchitis
- Pneumonia
- Bursitis
- Peripheral vascular disease
- Intermittent claudication (muscle pain with walking)
- Diabetic ulcers
- Thrombophlebitis

This is a very simple, highly effective therapy which addresses pathogens and mitochondrial dysfunction.

High-Dose Vitamin C

Vitamin C is considered an antioxidant but when doses upwards of 25 grams are administered intravenously over an hour and a half, vitamin C causes an oxidative response in the body.

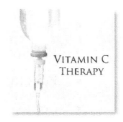

VITAMIN C
THERAPY

Therefore, this administration characteristically acts like the other oxidative therapies mentioned above and mimics what our own white blood cells do to fight infections.

Vitamin C is important for another reason as well.

Besides our white cells secreting hydrogen peroxide to reduce pathogens, white cells also do our housekeeping, by eating or phagocytizing debris and dead pathogens.

After the Zotzmann and UBI, huge numbers of dead bacteria flow back into our veins.

This does have the benefit of stimulating our immune system with an increase in the number of white blood cells and potentially their activity.

But if our white cells are to phagocytize all these dead organisms, they must be fed, and the primary nutrient they require is vitamin C.

Please note that before administering any IV high-dose vitamin C a person much first have a blood test called G6PD.

Nutrient IVs

As you know, every cell in the body requires nutrients to function optimally. This includes not only the cell's inner workings (nucleus, mitochondria, etc.) but the intricate make-up of the inner and outer membranes as well.

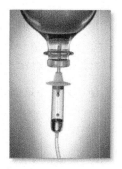

Nutritional IVs:

These IVs include C, all the B vitamins, various minerals and trace minerals which primarily address the cells' internal nutrient needs.

BiOcean

This product is imported from France.

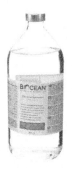

Deep ocean water is collected or harvested and then processed through a sophisticated cold-filtration system leaving all minerals and trace minerals intact.

In our Earth's history, it was once covered by waters rich in minerals and trace minerals and when the oceans receded, our soil was a repository for all these nutrients.

Most of them have become depleted from our soil and even if we consume organic foods, we are unlikely to receive the full spectrum of minerals and trace minerals our cells require to thrive.

Meyers Cocktail

This is a quick and simple means of delivering vitamin C, various minerals and B vitamins mixed with sterile water.

It is also called a Meyers Push since these ingredients are drawn into a 60cc syringe, rather than a large IV bag, and slowly injected into a vein.

The push takes about 5 to 10 minutes to complete.

Plaquex

The Plaquex formula has been used for over 55 years in about ¼ of the world's countries and was originally developed to resolve fatty embolus (plaque) during and after surgery.

Plaquex repairs and improves all our cellular membranes since ½ of their outer membrane is made up of phospholipids.

In the 1990s, its' therapeutic focus shifted to complement IV EDTA chelation therapy for circulatory and cardiovascular issues.

It has also been used as an anti-ageing therapy since many doctors observed their patients looking younger and feeling healthier after a course of Plaquex.

A healthier cell membrane allows increased waste excretion and increased uptake of vital nutrients.

Plaquex is designed to repair cell membranes that have been damaged by toxic substances, heavy metals, solvents and free radicals.

Plaquex repairs and reconditions the lining of blood vessels to improve circulation and oxygen delivery to tissues.

Anytime we improve circulation and the delivery of oxygen to cells, we are again back to correcting mitochondrial dysfunction.

Plaquex is an essential phospholipid formula containing Polyenyl Phosphatidyl Choline and is administered intravenously.

Its uses include the following:

- Improves lipid profile
- Improves liver function
- Decreases plaque in arteries
- Increases mental function
- Improves kidney function

This is a simple treatment that lasts about 90 minutes.

Plaquex is injected into a 250cc IV bag filled with sterile D5W, or Dextrose, and then delivered into any vein.

IVs For Liver & General Detoxification

Glutathione

This is given as a push from a syringe directly into the vein.

Glutathione is an antioxidant and helps to neutralize free radicals and improve the liver's ability to clear toxins from the blood.

Alpha Lipoic Acid

ALA improves mitochondrial activity and specifically helps to repair liver cells and to improve their function.

Lipoic acid is also an antioxidant and can potentiate the benefits of the IV vitamin C when administered afterwards.

IVs for Heavy Metal Toxins

For directly binding onto heavy metals there are three types of chelation therapies.

Chelation Therapy

Chelation is usually thought of for cardiac and circulatory issues. The form used is Disodium EDTA.

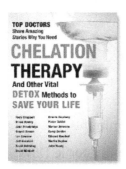

This has proven to be a very effective way to improve circulation by removing accumulated plaque on arterial walls.

It is a long IV, around three hours.

The benefits of Disodium EDTA chelation are amplified when done in conjunction with IV Plaquex mentioned above.

Another type of chelator is Calcium EDTA which is specific for binding to a variety of heavy metals including lead, aluminum, arsenic, cadmium and others.

This is a shorter IV, usually around 45 minutes.

The 3rd chelation solution is DMPS which is specific for mercury and requires about a half-hour.

All chelation IVs have vitamin C added to the mix.

All the chelation IVs require a few blood tests to check kidney function, a complete blood count and an iron panel.

The Kidney Function Blood Panel is used to determine the optimal concentration of each of the three chelating solutions.

For all the above we recommend specific supplements to support the pathways of detoxification and to ensure optimal mineral levels.

IVs for Drug & Chemical Withdrawal

Mitochondrial Function and NAD

Intravenous Nicotinamide Adenine Dinucleotide is the most effective means of detoxifying stored drug and chemical residues from within our cells.

NAD feeds or activates our mitochondria, which increases the production of ATP. Cells can then actively transport and excrete any chemical or toxic residue from within.

NAD IV therapy is our first choice for every client who wants to discontinue their prescription or drug.

This approach is far superior to any rehab center in the world.

NAD is at the core of our drug addiction program.

You can learn more about the program we offer by visiting our other site, https://ivnaddrugaddictions.com/

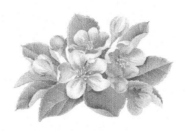

CONSTITUTIONAL THERAPIES
FOR RECOVERY

During my last year at the University of Natural Medicine, I spent three days preceptoring with an ND, Dr. Harold Dick.

He had a small clinic in eastern Washington, specializing in what was called Constitutional Hydrotherapy, the use of hot and cold compresses to the chest, abdomen and back.

This therapy originates from another ND, Dr. Carroll, who travelled extensively throughout Europe, to learn about the use of water therapies in a number of clinics.

Carroll distilled what he observed, and developed a way of improving lymphatic drainage in order to stimulate this important pathway of detoxification.

Lymph is a fluid which bathes all our cells and consists of proteins, white blood cells, toxins, bacteria, hormones, fats, salts and water.

It is this liquid through which nutrients, toxins and hormones pass through from the blood on their way to cells. Since this fluid resides just outside our cells, if we are working with cellular detoxification, we must ensure that our lymph is moving in order to transport these toxic residues away from cells and tissues, which are then dumped into our blood stream.

Lymph is likely the least considered concern when it come to a cause of ill-health.

Anyway, Dr. Dick would see each new patient to determine if they had any food allergies, and these foods would need to be avoided during the hydrotherapy treatments.

Then their treatments would begin, twice daily.

He told each patient that he could not predict how many treatments would be needed.

So the question was, how did he determine when a patient didn't need any further treatments.

Before each hydrotherapy session, Dr. Dick would listen to their heart with a stethoscope.

I asked what he was listening for.

He was a very simple man, taking time between patients to work on his car and to smoke a cigarette.

'It's like listening to a truck, struggling to make it up a steep grade. It sounds like their heart is struggling.'

'When they no longer need the treatment, the heart sounds like it's now purring downhill.'

I didn't think this analogy sounded very medical, but I respected his approach.

Thinking more about it, he made sense, because lymph fluid drains back into the circulatory system just above the heart.

The heart is a very sensitive organ, and any toxins cause a great deal of stress upon the heart.

So, if the lymph is clean and most toxins have been cleared, it would make sense that the heart would 'purr' as he said.

I thought my visit would be simply observational, but he told me that the only way to know and to understand the therapy's benefits, would be to experience it.

So, for three day, twice daily, I received the treatment.

When I returned to school, another student helped me to continue with this therapy.

During this time, I experience a great deal of mental clarity and an increase in physical energy.

Such a simple concept, that no matter what condition a person is suffering from, no matter what the diagnosis, their health will improve.

With this guiding principle, that certain therapies will help everyone to recovery their health no matter what their condition is, they can be included under this general heading of 'Constitutional Therapies.'

Remember, the absence of symptoms indicates optimal cellular function, and that symptoms reflect a lowering of cellular function.

There are many reasons for this decline in function, which was already covered; lack of vital nutrients, toxins and low grade, chronic, systemic infections.

If we consider ways to improve health, they must increase cellular function and improve the pathways of detoxification.

Remember, detoxification starts at the cellular levels, and when the cell becomes strong enough to excrete these toxins, they will travel from the interior of cells to the exterior, and into the lymph.

From there they travel through the lymph into the bloodstream, and then removed through the kidneys and liver.

From the liver they enter the gallbladder, and then into the intestines.

So, if we can improve any of these pathways, the person's health will also improve.

Please also recall that many toxic residues are stored in fat cells just under the skin, called the subdermal fat layer.

The following is a list of 'Constitutional Therapies to improve overall vitality.

Lymphatic or Constitutional Hydrotherapy

Here is an outline of how I was taught by Dr. Dick to administer this therapy.

You lie on your back on a massage table, undressed from the waist up and covered with wool blankets.

The blankets are then pulled down to uncover the chest and abdomen, and a moist, thick hot compress is placed to cover from just under the neck to the pubic bone and to the sides of the chest and abdomen.

Once the compress is in place, blankets are adjusted to cover the hot compress and tucked tightly around the sides of the waist, chest and shoulders.

This heating compress remains for five minutes.

So, what is the body's response to this hot compress?

You know that any heat applied to the skin causes a reddening since blood is moved into the small capillary blood vessels just under the skin.

This reaction is because heat causes an increase in the metabolism of cells > then cells give off more waste (CO_2) >

this increases acidity > causing increase in the diameter of blood vessels > resulting in increased blood flow > increased delivery of oxygen > improved removal of CO2 and cellular waste.

But something else is going on here which is just as important.

Over the entire body we have dermatomes which run in parallel lines along our skin. Each dermatome covers a distinct skin area of the body.

When a dermatome on the skin is heated its corresponding internal organs, connected through the nerves of the spinal column, react in a similar way with increased blood flow.

So, heat placed on the skin say at dermatome 7 and 9 will cause the dilation of blood vessels within the liver.

DERMATOMES

With the application of a hot compress over the chest and abdomen all the underlying organs will be filled with fresh blood causing increased oxygen, increased delivery of nutrients and the removal of metabolic waste and toxins.

By the way, this hot compress is also very relaxing.

After five minutes, another hot compress is laid on top of the 1st hot compress, turned over and then is quickly replaced by a cold compress covering the same area of the chest and abdomen.

This cold compress remains for 10 minutes.

Now what is happening?

The body's **initial** reaction to cold is the opposite of heat.

Basically, the blood vessels just under the skin constrict which drives the blood deep into the core of the body.

This same initial reaction is occurring to the internal organs as well since the dermatomes are sending a chilling or constricting message.

So, the reaction at the internal organ level is constriction, like the wringing out of a sponge.

This is the immediate reaction to cold (constriction) but then there's a **secondary** reaction because the body will redirect blood to the skin to warm the cold compress.

Over the 10-minute application of the cold compress to the chest and abdomen, warm blood is shunted to the skin and to all the internal organs.

This pumping action of blood flowing back and forth to the skin and in and out of the organs has many benefits including purification.

This approach of alternating hot and cold also increases the activity of what's called the 'lymphatic pump.'

To activate this pump even further, we use a sine wave machine which causes a gentle contraction and relaxation of the muscles along the spine and over the center section of the abdomen.

After the hot and cold compresses to the chest and abdomen, you then turn onto your stomach and the same procedure, 5 minutes of the hot compress followed by 10 minutes of the cold compress, is repeated.

This is the premier therapy for not only lymphatic drainage but also improving digestive issues, blood sugar dysregulation and liver, gall bladder and kidney drainage.

This treatment requires about 50 minutes from start to finish.

We recommend this treatment be done as often as possible, even every day if you can, depending upon your level of toxicity.

Saunas to the Rescue

I sincerely believe that if saunas were incorporated into our lifestyle, we would not be witnessing such a rapid decline in the health of our population.

Of course, this belief is based upon environmental toxins and the biofilm produced by pathogens being two primary causes of illness.

Even though the wide array of toxins and chemical residues find their way into various tissues, fat cells are the primary repository.

There's a layer of fat beneath the skin called the subdermal fat layer. Getting toxic residues out of this layer is accomplished through perspiration.

This is why sauna therapy is essential for detoxification and purification since we prefer to have toxins excreted through the skin rather than entering our lymph and blood.

The Benefits of Sauna

For centuries saunas have been used by various cultures for purification, relaxation, spiritual rites and connecting with nature.

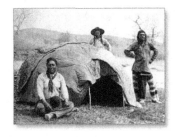

Yet how often do we sweat?

We go from our air-conditioned homes to our air-conditioned cars.

Many of us do not have a job that requires much physical exertion and therefore we do not sweat.

We use antiperspirants and apply skin creams which leave residues that block the pores of our sweat glands.

So, saunas, if we are to improve our health, must become a part of our lifestyle.

The Sauna Experience

How our body is stimulated to sweat <u>does</u> make a difference with how well toxins are excreted.

During the sauna experience you should feel completely relaxed. This means that perspiring during exercise will not be as effective with purification when compared with relaxing in the sauna.

We want blood to flow to our skin and not necessarily to our muscles.

This is key. The more relaxed our muscles are the easier blood will flow from the core of our bodies to the surface. This easier flow keeps the heart calm and maintains a lower heart rate and blood pressure.

This also has to do with the Autonomic Nervous System because perspiring while relaxed will improve the parasympathetic branch while reducing sympathetic stimulation.

We prefer the dry heat sauna rather than infrared since IR penetrates deeper into tissues, it can trigger the release of toxins into the blood stream rather than externally through the skin.

Ozone Sauna

Besides the purification benefits of hot steam, when ozone flows into the sauna chamber it penetrates through moist skin and into the small capillaries.

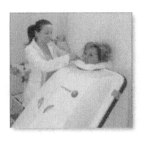

One benefit of ozone is its anti-pathogenic properties. In other words, it will kill and inhibit the growth of bacteria, viruses and molds.

Ozone is used in medicine around the world in clinics and hospitals as a standalone therapy for decreasing pathogens and increasing oxygenation of tissues.

The time in this sauna depends upon the person's tolerance to heat. We can adjust the temperature inside the sauna to make it more comfortable, so people can remain longer.

The usual time is anywhere between 30 and 50 minutes.

During this sauna, a person can step into an adjacent shower to cool off. The cold shower will amplify the benefits since alternating hot and cold will activate greater detoxification.

After the ozone sauna the person takes a warm shower to remove oils and toxins from the skin, so they are not reabsorbed through the skin back into the body.

Walk-in Dry Sauna

Our walk-in sauna is private unless you request another to join you.

There is plenty of room to lie down and to relax.

The primary advantage of the walk-in sauna is comfort and being able to easily alternate between hot and cold.

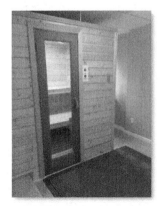

Next to the sauna is a shower.

Now if you remember the benefits of the alternating hot and cold compresses with the Lymphatic, or Constitutional Hydrotherapy, you will understand why we have located a shower so close to the sauna.

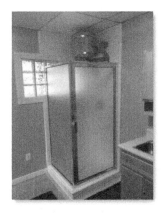

After working up a good sweat and you sense the body would like a refreshing cool rinse you step out of the sauna and into the shower closet.

The cool or cold shower, depending on your tolerance, is not only refreshing but stimulates circulation, corresponding dermatomal organs below the skin, and your mitochondria.

Some studies say that cold also stimulates the release of stem cells.

Maybe you have heard of Cryotherapy, the use of cold, either sitting in a cold room or lying in cold water.

This cold shower also allows people to remain in the sauna for a longer period of time.

We recommend going back and forth between the sauna and the shower, always starting with the sauna and finishing with cold.

So, after cycles of hot sauna and cold shower, you finish with a lukewarm shower to remove all oils and residues from the skin with a chemical free soap.

The Bemer

Dr. Alfred Pischinger, MD (1899-1982) from Austria was the first scientist to describe the regulation of the Extracellular Matrix (ECM) and stated that health and disease is determined by the state or quality of this Matrix tissue.

This Matrix includes the lymph system, or lymph fluid, AND the fluid (blood) in the capillaries of the circulatory system adjacent to the lymph.

If this Matrix is clean and free of toxins, then the person will most likely remain healthy.

If it is unclean and more like a swamp, then the person will most likely become ill.

If the Matrix is running like a stream, then toxins excreted by cells will be easily cleared away.

So besides clearing this swamp with Lymphatic Hydrotherapy, what else can be done?

Let's talk about the capillaries, our smallest blood vessels, which are part of this Matrix.

As arteries become smaller (arterioles) and smaller we finally come to the tiny capillaries through which red blood cells flow through in order to deliver oxygen and to carry away waste.

Before each capillary is a tiny muscle called the pre-capillary sphincter.

If this muscle is tight then blood flow is restricted.

Red cells are not able to pass through this tight sphincter into the capillary. Even the flow of serum, the liquid part of the blood which carries nutrients, is restricted.

What if we could relax this tiny muscle?

This would help to increase mitochondrial function because of improved oxygen delivery, increased availability of nutrients and improved clearing of toxic residues.

A German company was given the task of preventing chronic illnesses in their older population to reduce government spending on health care.

They developed the Bemer which emits what they call micro-Tesla frequencies which specifically relax this pre-capillary sphincter.

This is normally an eight-minute treatment with the person lying on a full-length mat which is emitting these frequencies.

We normally use the Bemer before each IV therapy to enhance the delivery of nutrients to tissues.

Colon Hydrotherapy

A future chapter on Gut Health addresses several issues related to digestion, assimilation and harmful waste products from bacteria and parasites in the gut which are detrimental to cellular and mitochondrial function.

The gut is one avenue the body uses to expel toxins and must therefore be considered during purification.

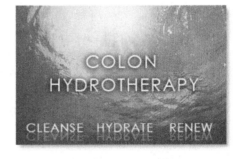

When toxins are metabolized and filtered from the blood by the liver, they first pass through the gall bladder on their way to the small intestines.

Once these toxins reach the gut, they must then travel the entire length of the intestines which is about 20 feet.

The faster we can move these toxins through the gut the less likely they will be absorbed back into the body.

Colon hydrotherapy is an excellent way to support detoxification because it assists the body to excrete toxins and takes a great strain off the liver and gall bladder to deal with the recycling of toxins.

During a purification program, as toxins are being released from cells and the lymph is dumping toxins into the blood stream, a person can feel unwell, what is sometimes called a Herx Reaction or a 'healing crisis.'

This is a perfect time to implement Colon Hydrotherapy.

The Procedure

During a series of Colon Hydrotherapy treatments, it is important to increase fiber rich foods, primarily raw vegetables, as well as fresh juices prepared from low glycemic vegetables.

Fiber will help in the process of scouring away old fecal material and will also bind toxic residues.

Our favorite soil-based probiotic should also be taken during this series to recolonize the gut with beneficial bacteria.

There are two types of colon hydrotherapy units.

One is called the 'closed system' which we used to use, and the other is the 'open system.'

Our unit is referred to as Angel of Waters Colon Hydrotherapy unit, which is a gravity-fed open design, used in clinics and hospitals around the world.

It is the safest, simplest and most effective solution for irrigating the colon, to remove impacted fecal and mucoid plaque.

When a client is comfortably positioned, a thin rectal nozzle is inserted into the rectum, about 1 ½ inches.

A gentle flow of gravity fed, 98-100 degree, filtered water begins.

Water flowing into the colon initiates peristalsis, or movement of the muscles surrounding the colon, and the patient responds by relieving water and waste repeatedly over the course of the 35-45 minute session.

The progressive irrigation and hydration which starts in the rectum, progresses through the entire colon, from the descending, across the transverse and down the ascending sections, breaking apart waste matter to achieve the complete evacuation of the colon.

This is a very gentle and effective therapy.

Our colon hydro-therapist is fully trained and certified with years of experience.

She will also begin with an initial consultation to review your symptoms, nutrition and supplements to be sure you receive the most benefits from this purification therapy.

Multi-Wave Oscillator (MWO)

Medicine sees humans through the lens of biology, the study of life and living organisms including physical structure, chemical processes, molecular interactions and physiological mechanisms.

There are limitations to this perspective since we are more than just the sum of our parts.

Physics, especially quantum mechanics, sees the world through the lens of subatomic particles, both wave-like and particle-like, which is applicable to molecules, atoms, electrons, protons and other subatomic particles, of which we are composed.

Thus, we are more than meets the eye and for that matter, all our senses.

Might illness originate deep into the interior of cells, into other worlds not considered or comprehended by modern medicine?

Are there existing therapies which can benefit our health through frequencies which positively correct any disturbance in the disequilibrium of our energetic 'field?'

Yes, and the approach must be to increase the oscillation or vibration of all our cells, and this is the primary function or result of entering ourselves within the field of a very wide range of oscillating frequencies.

According to the scientist who developed the MWO unit, George Lakhovsky, as these frequencies are broadcast, every cell will find its specific resonant frequency, resulting in an increase is cellular vibration and health.

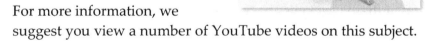

Thus, we have another 'Constitutional Therapy' which will improve a person's health no matter what their condition.

For more information, we suggest you view a number of YouTube videos on this subject.

Juice Fasting

There are at least three reasons why juicing is beneficial.

The 1st is that juices provide a broad spectrum of enzymes and nutrients which nourish our cells and address the first primary cause of illness, nutritional deficiencies.

The 2nd is that, because our cells are receiving more nutrients, our mitochondria begin to function better. More ATP production increases the excretion of toxic residues from within our cells.

The 3rd is that, if low glycemic vegetables are used to make juice then the body will call upon fat cells for free fatty acids which will indirectly causes the release of toxins.

Juice fasting is much less extreme than water and sometimes I favor this approach, since it provides plenty of nutrients which water does not.

For many people I recommend drinking juices throughout the day and to have a specific meal at night. This will slow down the detoxification a bit and people often need some form of protein to aid in the metabolism and excretion of toxins.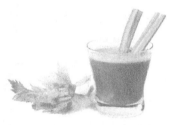

Of course, when it comes to vegetables, they MUST be organic.

Think about preparing and eating a salad, made from the same amount you'd need to make an eight-ounce glass of juice. Likely you could never finish it because this is a lot of vegetables.

So, if these vegetables have been sprayed, you are consuming a lot of chemical residues.

I know the entire procedure of juicing, from making a list, shopping, washing, juicing and cleaning up can be overwhelming.

And in some months of the year the availability of organic produce is slim.

There is a very high-quality vegetable powder product we recommend which is an excellent alternative to fresh juice.

Their dehydration process uses very little heat and thus protects enzymes and nutrients from oxidation, to remain active and viable.

Intermittent Fasting

As a reminder, another way to help your cells detoxify is intermittent fasting using diluted fresh lemon juice.

This approach works well for people whose nutrient status is acceptable, meaning they've been on a good nutritional program and don't have a lot of nutritional deficiencies.

So, here are two examples of intermittent fasting that work well for most people.

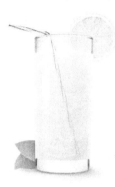

Drink a glass of water with ½ of a squeezed organic lemon. If there are blood sugar issues, specifically low blood sugar or hypoglycemia, you may be asked to add a bit of maple syrup.

This is all you have during the morning until lunch.

If you finish dinner around 6pm and drink only the lemonade until noon the next day this would be an 18 hour fast.

During this time, you've helped your cells to go through some purification and if you are feeling well at noon you can even extend the lemonade drink until dinner.

Now you've done a 24 hour fast.

Remember, if you experience unpleasant symptoms such as headaches, nausea, fatigue and muscle aches and pains, then this is a good thing.

What?

These symptoms are a sign that your body is going through a detox or purification at the cellular level.

It could also mean that your pathways of detoxification are not working well, and you'll need to support these pathways with some purification therapies and some specific liver and kidney herbs.

Contrary to the beliefs of other practitioners, I believe the evening meal is most important. Some believe that a light dinner is preferable, so the body doesn't have to deal with digestion during sleep but in many cases I disagree.

Many people have sleep issues primarily due to blood sugar dysregulation. They slip into hypoglycemia (low blood sugar) when sleeping and wake up in a 'fight or flight' mode due to increased levels of adrenaline.

This relates to adrenal fatigue.

There are certainly other causes for insomnia.

I also believe that the body is very active during sleep with repair and preparing for the next day.

Providing the body with plenty of nutrients at dinnertime is very important.

In some cases, I might not recommend this, and to shift the most important meal to the morning, and this is determined by blood tests for fasting glucose and the HA1c which indicates how well a person is regulating their blood sugar.

Final Words

To summarize, no matter what condition you are suffering from, you will definitely benefit from any of these therapies.

It is one thing to have had a consultation with Dr. Haskell, and to have discovered some underlying issues for your condition.

This discussion likely ended with a specific program to address these causes.

To potentiate and enhance this program, 'Constitutional Therapies' are an important adjunct, meaning they will complement and accelerate the recovery of your health and vitality.

In part, to actively engage in these therapies as often as possible, is your responsibility.

Consider the following as a weekly routine;

- Myers Push (vitamin C & other nutrients) 20 minutes

- Bemer (open the matrix) 8 minutes

- MWO (increase cellular activity) 15-20 minutes

- Sauna (detox & lymph drainage) 45-50 minutes

The total time is about an hour and a half at a cost of around $110.

Maybe it's time to make time and form new healthy habits.

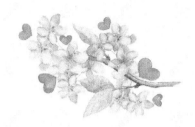

GUT HEALTH

We cannot speak about removing toxins from the body and correcting nutritional deficiencies without touching upon the environment of our intestinal tract.

We can select the highest quality nutrient dense foods but if we cannot digest them completely then a portion of these nutrients pass through us and never enter the body.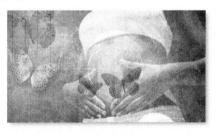

If barriers to assimilating these nutrients through the delicate lining of our small intestines are present, then the same issue of delivery exists.

If the population of beneficial bacteria have been reduced by the overuse of antibiotics then the nutrients, especially the B vitamins and vitamin K which are produced by these symbiotic organisms, will not be received either.

If we have an overgrowth of unfriendly bacteria and yeast in the gut, their metabolic waste products will interfere with assimilating nutrients and will seep into the body, creating a variety of physical and mental symptoms.

If there are parasites, and most people have them, not only will they consume nutrients from your food, but their waste products will also negatively impact your health.

Toxins produced by bacteria, fungi and parasites also enter the cells that line the gut and disrupt their function. Many of these cells are part of our Enteric Nervous System which is responsible for producing various hormones we associate with our brain, like serotonin.

Then there's the 'Leaky Gut' syndrome where the lining of the small intestine is breaking down. This primarily happens from chronic bowel inflammation and various medications including non-steroidal anti-inflammatories (NSAIDs).

With this condition, a person will experience allergic type reactions to foods because the immune system is in a hyper-reactive state due to the passing of food particles through the gut which should remain within the confines of the small intestines.

So, as you can see, we've got other causes of symptoms at work here.

- Nutritional deficiencies from digestion and assimilation issues.
- Toxins from pathogenic waste products entering the body and all our cells.

The function and environment (ecology) of this tube that runs through us has as much influence upon our health as our external environment.

If our gut is messed up, how can we ever expect to get well?

To remedy gut issues there are several approaches:

- Help the body to digest food more thoroughly.
    - This can require digestive enzymes such as

80

capsules of hydrochloric acid, betaine and pepsin and possibly bile salts if a gall bladder issue exists.

   o   Eat simply and limit your meal to two foods.

- Consider the possibility of Candida lining the gut which impedes assimilation. Candida results from the overuse of antibiotics and consuming a lot of simple carbohydrates and sugars.

- Replenish beneficial bacteria starting with a 'soil' probiotic first.

- Determine if there's an overgrowth of bacteria in the gut, known as SIBO. There is a breath test for this.

- If you suspect the lining of the intestines has been damaged, it may be useful to get a blood test to confirm.

   o   Cyrex Labs offers the best test for determining Leaky Gut.

- Go through a gut purification program which among other things includes Colon Hydrotherapy.

Bacterial Flora & Weight Gain

For those of you struggling to lose weight you might find this section of the chapter interesting.

Could an imbalance of the microbial inhabitants of our intestines be another underlying cause of weight gain, and thus an increase in the storage of toxic residues?

In 1950 a team of scientists discovered that adding antibiotics to livestock feed accelerated weight gain in animals.

At that time, this industry was using conventional livestock supplements such as fish meal from Japan and cod liver oil from Norway.

These were expensive compared with synthetic antibiotics so the transition from 'food' supplements to antibiotics for livestock was a financial decision.

Today we think that antibiotics are primarily used to decrease the rate of infections of animals living in crowded quarters, yet their original use was to increase weight.

Today, of the 40 million pounds (wow… 20,000 tons) of antibiotics produced in the US, about 29 million pounds are being used in the meat industry.

Why antibiotics cause primarily gain in fat tissue is still unclear.

Maybe the reasons are as follows;

- Antibiotics causes a change in the animal's intestinal flora
- Yeast or fungal issues in the gut rise
- Fungal waste products enter the animal from the gut
- This waste enters primarily fat cells
- Mitochondrial activity in fat cells slows as a result
- This lowered activity causes fat cells to store more fat and less able to excrete fat

Symbiosis: Mutually Beneficial Relationship

There exists a natural balance among all the beneficial types of microbes in the gut with an estimated population being over 100 trillion. Amazing that these beneficial gut microbes outnumber the cells of our body.

They protect us from pathogens, provide us with nutrients and help regulate our immune system.

Alterations or a decline in these microbes have been linked with many gastrointestinal disorders, diabetes, certain cancers and obesity.

If we are going to regain our health, lose weight and free our bodies from toxins, we must understand how these microbes came to inhabit our gut as well as the causes for their decline.

In the fetal stage, our intestinal tract is sterile meaning there are no living microbes in our gut.

When birthed we pass through the vaginal canal where microbes are introduced. When breast fed, we add additional microbes from the skin of our mother and through breast milk.

Their population rapidly rises until, by the first or second year of life, our intestines are teaming with these symbiotic microbes.

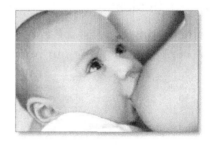

Luckily breast feeding is on the rise from 22% in 1972 to 82% in 2013. Human breast milk including the colostrum contains more than 700 species of beneficial bacteria which colonize the digestive system.

Yet cesarean sections which bypass this vaginal birth canal have risen from 5% in 1960 to about 30% today. This means that around three in ten people are deficient in these life supporting microbes.

Then there's the use of antibiotics which disrupt the balance of our innate flora.

Before the mid-1900s we didn't have penicillin.

Yet these days antibiotics are overused and abused.

Before the age of two, 70% of children are prescribed antibiotics with an average of about two prescriptions per child.

This disrupts the population of good bacteria in the gut and leads to an imbalance between two specific categories of bacteria called Firmicutes and Bacteroidetes.

In mice and a few human studies, fat gain is seen when the Bacteroidetes in the gut are low.

To reestablish this type of bacteria we recommend the use of a 'soil' based probiotic.

Since our objective is to get toxins out of fat cells, and of course other cells as well, we must focus on weight loss and thus the need to implant these soil bacteria into our intestines.

Remediating or reestablishing the microflora of the gut is at the core of recovering our innate health and well-being.

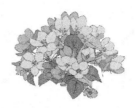

TOXINS: THE 2ND CAUSE OF ILLNESS

If you want to completely recover your health and prevent future health issues, it is important to understand the insidious nature of environmental toxins.

You can use all our therapies to recover your health but if you remain complacent about your exposure to toxins, you'll eventually be right back to where you started.

We will therefore uncover a number of toxins, how they can potentially impact your health and what you can do to avoid them.

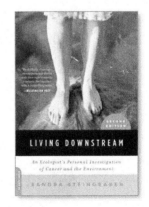

Thousands of research articles have been published by reputable journals proving the harmful effects of chemicals in our environment.

Two books I recommend which consolidate this research using stories and clinical pearls are *Living Downstream* by Sandra Steingraber, PhD, and *Detoxify or Die* by Dr. Sherry Rogers, MD.

Environmental Toxins

During our entire lifetime we have been exposed to a wide range of toxins in our environment, many of which have been labeled or identified as being harmful to humans.

Yet with the financial clout of corporations and government lobbyists, the unregulated and irresponsible use of highly toxic chemicals still prevails.

These toxins enter us through our skin, our lungs and our mouths.

Most of us think toxins are outside our homes. We don't realize that indoor household toxins reach very high levels because our homes are sealed in the warmer and cooler seasons resulting in a recycling effect.

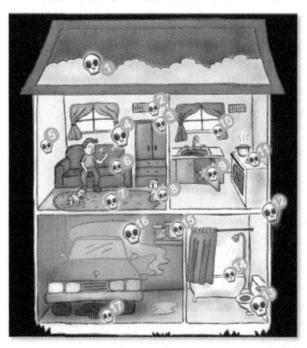

The most common toxins we breathe in the home are radon, the volatile organic compounds outgassing from our furnishings and carpets, chemicals in cleaning solutions, and insecticides.

The most common toxins that penetrate our skin are found in cleaning solutions, hair dyes, cosmetics, deodorants, antibacterial soaps and skin care products.

The most common toxins we consume are preservatives, colorings, chlorine and petrochemical residues, plastics in bottles and the lining of cans, and pesticides and herbicides sprayed on our produce.

When low level toxins enter and accumulate in our tissues vague symptoms may begin to appear. Becoming aware of these symptoms is one way our innate wisdom is trying to communicate to us that something is wrong.

It is trying to get our attention, to wake us up to the fact that something is not right, that something in our environment or in our food is causing us harm.

It calls out, 'Wake up,' through sinus issues, digestive complaints, asthma, joint pains, fatigue, nausea, insomnia, depression or just not feeling right.

Yet most people don't get the message and often turn to over-the-counter medications, supplements and herbs to relieve their symptoms.

So, the question is, 'How can we discover and identify these harmful toxins that are odorless, tasteless and insidious?'

Our EPA & FDA

Most chemicals we are exposed to have not undergone any toxicological studies by our EPA (Environmental Protection Agency) and FDA (Federal Drug Administration), which admit that almost all the chemicals manufactured in the

United States are poisonous to humans.

For some bizarre reason they are considered 'safe' if used in moderation.

The term 'safe' assumes that dangerous chemicals delivered in small seemingly harmless amounts are acceptable because they will pass through us as if unnoticed.

Yet it's been proven that when these toxins enter our bodies, they are not completely eliminated yet stored in various tissues.

Our EPA even performed fat biopsies on cadavers which revealed a wide array of residues from petrochemical products including pesticides such as DDT, herbicides and BPA from plastics to name but a few.

From this study it's obvious that we do not completely metabolize and excrete environmental toxins.

They accumulate in various tissues, especially fat cells, which will eventually lead to physical and mental symptoms.

Living on this polluted planet, everyone has stored toxins.

On another note, for those of you who believe in inherited genetic illnesses, several studies have shed light upon the debate between genetics vs. environmental toxins.

Studies out of Norway and Sweden examined the health of adults who were adopted as children.

Researchers asked the question, 'Have these adoptees developed health issues similar to their birth parents or their foster parents.'

Turns out the later was true and likely points to the family's nutritional habits and environmental exposures.

The evolution of genetic research has morphed into

epigenetics which is the study of how environmental factors influence the expression of our genetic heritage.

A Case of Environmental Toxicity

Around two years ago a gentleman presented with a bizarre set of symptoms.

Up until the last three days his health had been fine, but now he complained of recent headaches, insomnia and so weak that he could barely get out of bed.

His most troublesome symptom was not being able to urinate unless he sat in a bathtub of hot water.

I told him there must be some reasons or causes for his symptoms. I suspected his environment.

After our consult we administered a nutrient vitamin C IV and a 45-minute ozone sauna session.

Vitamin C supported his immune system and addressed his adrenal fatigue.

Saunas helped his body to eliminate toxic residues through the skin.

He called 3 hours later to say he felt 75% better and felt the sauna had helped the most.

To me this confirmed that his environment was the culprit, so we set up a time for me to visit his home the following day.

Here's what we discovered.

- The living room in his rented condo had veneer floors. This room faced west, and the hot afternoon sun was likely causing elevated temperatures in his condo resulting in the outgassing of volatile organic compounds from the veneer. He mentioned he was never home in the afternoons and with windows closed this room was sweltering hot.

- We discovered mold behind the washer dryer units located next to his bedroom.

- The bathtub in his primary bathroom and the sink in his second bathroom were never used so the 'U' joints in the plumbing were dry allowing hydrogen sulfide gas to rise from the sewer.

- Pesticide cartridges were found under the stove and behind the refrigerator.

- Polyester (plastic) carpeting in his bedroom was also subjected to the high afternoon heat resulting in the outgassing of other chemicals.

So, he remediated everything he could and from that day forward all windows were kept open to allow fresh air to circulate.

He continued daily saunas for about two weeks even though most of his symptoms were better with 48 hours.

He gave notice and moved within the month.

As I said before, symptoms are a true blessing and communicate to us that insults must be investigated and rectified.

What do you think our medical system would have done with a case like his?

When we come to the aid of our innate physician by investigating and removing causes and at the same time cleanse impurities through purification therapies the restoration of our health is inevitable.

Paracelsus: Physician and Alchemist

Paracelsus was considered the father of toxicology.

He stated, 'All substances are poisons. There is none which is not a poison. The right dose differentiates a poison from a remedy.'

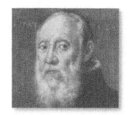

Yet can we say there is a safe dose for all the man-made chemicals such as herbicides, pesticides, PCBs and the like?

Not really, and their harmful effects depend upon two factors; the quantity we are exposed to and the body's ability to neutralize and excrete them.

So, given the fact that we are exposed to more than 80,000 chemicals produced in the United States, most of which have not been tested for their 'toxicity potential', how can we protect ourselves and support our body's excretory pathways?

Pharmaceutical & OTC Drug Toxins

In the chapter on mitochondria I briefly mentioned mitochondrial dysfunction due to prescriptions and OTC medications.

Because of their detrimental effects upon mitochondria, I consider these synthetics to be another insult to human health.

All side effects listed for any drug are the direct result of their disrupting effects upon mitochondria function.

And the reason why drugs, especially the psycho-pharmaceuticals, are so difficult to wean off of is because they leave the affected cells unable to function optimally, and thus the need to continue taking the drug.

So, the way out of an 'addiction' to a medication would be the following;

- Nourish the mitochondria to increase their activity. This helps our cells to do what they are designed to do and simultaneously enables them to excrete drug and toxic residues.

- Use IVs that promote mitochondria function such as NAD, Lipoic Acid and Acetyl L-Carnitine.

- Use purification therapies to excrete drug residues through the skin, lymph, liver, kidney and colon.

- Address the three primary causes of mental and physical symptoms, which likely existed in the first place when a psychopharmaceutical was first prescribed.

- Improve the pathways of detoxification so the excreted drug residues will more easily be eliminated from the body.

I believe it is a crime when a person has been prescribed a long-term medication without thoroughly investigating the causes for their symptoms.

I am sure there are times when this approach is necessary but a thorough biochemical and hormonal investigation must be the first step.

Let's take depression as one example.

I have seen hundreds of clients suffering from depression. Every one of them had several underlying biochemical, hormonal, environmental and pathogenic causes.

All these causes must be investigated BEFORE a prescription is offered;

- Suboptimal thyroid hormones

- Autoimmune Hashimoto's

- Estrogen dominance with low progesterone

- Very low vitamin D levels

- Adrenal exhaustion with low cortisol production

- Vacillating blood sugar levels

- Low cholesterol intake, cholesterol being the vital nutrient required for the production of all steroid hormones

- Low B12, B6 and other nutrient deficiencies due to various causes including oral contraceptives

- Active tooth abscess undiagnosed by their dentist

- Insomnia due to blood sugar fluctuations and low progesterone

- Chronic viral infections

- Small intestinal bacteria overgrowth

- Chronic yeast infections in the gut

- Parasites

- Poor absorption of nutrients due to hydrochloric acid deficiencies

- Low protein diets

- Permeable gut leading to autoimmune conditions with elevated antibodies

- Mold sensitivities

And the list goes on and on.

Dirty Electricity

Strong electromagnetic fields are known stressors to all the cells of the body and brain. Some people are highly sensitive to even low levels of EMFs and are referred to as 'Electromagnetic Hypersensitives' or EHS.

In general, I don't believe that EMFs by themselves are enough to cause illness in the majority of people but when combined with many other threats and toxins, EMFs just become another contributing factor.

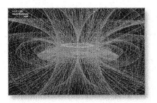 There is so much I could say about the harmful effects of EMFs, but I suggest watching a video given by Dr. Rhoda Alale, PhD.

She is a dynamic and passionate speaker and relates a very personal story about how EMFs affected her health and that of her son.

One of her best YouTube videos can be found by searching her name plus the acronym CHEUSE.

There are many EMF meters on the market for checking electrical outlets, microwave ovens, computers, lights and cell phones.

There are simple methods for grounding, to reduce the EMF load on your body.

I have also seen hypersensitive people have heavy metal issues such as lead, mercury, cadmium and others.

Dental metal fillings and metal implants likely increase our sensitivity.

Cosmetics? Oh, No!

We don't usually think of the skin as a semi-permeable membrane, but fat soluble, petrochemical based cosmetics and skin care products are absorbed through the skin into the body.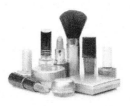

All cosmetics, whether it's lipsticks, creams, moisturizers or nail polish have solvents which facilitate rapid penetration of ingredients through the skin.

Lip gloss and lipsticks are not only absorbed through the skin but enter the mouth and are swallowed.

Because ingredients in lipsticks include solvents they pass through the delicate lining of the gut and carry with them whatever other chemicals are in the lipstick.

These solvents when swallowed also break down the 'glue' that maintains the integrity of the cells that line the intestines. Solvents are thus a contributing factor for what's called 'leaky gut.'

It may be difficult to comprehend but some cosmetic ingredients are classified as xenobiotics (carcinogenic contaminants).

Some lipstick and cosmetic products even contain heavy metals such as lead.

Common solvents are ethanol (usually made from corn, wheat and sugar cane), denatured alcohol, benzyl alcohol and isopropyl alcohol.

Ethanol has been shown to cause cell death (apoptosis) by damaging organelles (mitochondria) inside cells.

Some solvents are more benign such as Cetearyl alcohol and stearyl alcohol which are extracted from coconut oils.

The primary issue with cosmetics is that manufacturers are not required by law to list ingredients since they are not classified as a food for consumption even though they are absorbed into the body when applied to the skin and lips.

So why take the risk?

Why be naïve, thinking these products are harmless?

There are cosmetic companies using pure, natural ingredients in their manufacturing because there is a market for people knowledgeable about the toxins and endocrine disrupting chemicals found in cosmetics.

There's one company supplying cosmetics made from chemical free, wild crafted ingredients and can be found at AnnMarieGianni.com.

There's a saying, 'If you wouldn't eat what you are putting on your skin then don't use it.'

Fluoride

The question is, as with any chemical that has the potential to cause illness, 'What is a safe dose or exposure?'

Every scientist agrees that fluoride is toxic to humans yet few of them agree on what amount is safe.

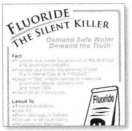

Then the question is, 'What are the potential benefits of fluoride and do they outweigh the harmful effects?'

This controversy around adding fluoride to our municipal water has existed since the 1950's.

Most people believe the reason for using fluoride is to reduce cavities. Yet in 1999 the Center for Disease Control admitted that the main dental benefit of fluoride is its use topically or orally and not when ingested.

The largest study ever, 39,000 children, was conducted between the years 1986 and 1987. It found that when comparing the teeth of those drinking fluoridated water with those who did not there was only 0.6 of one tooth surface improvement with the children drinking fluoridated water.

This benefit is miniscule and should not justify pouring fluoride into the water supply of every metropolitan household.

Does it make sense that fluoride, a known toxic chemical, should be blindly disseminated like this?

Fluoride is a hazardous waste product from various manufacturers including nuclear power plants. This waste cannot be legally dumped into streams, lakes or oceans and cannot be deposited in the earth.

But it can be sold as a product.

And who is buying it? Our water treatment plants.

We all know about dental fluorosis, the white mottling of teeth from excess fluoride but there are negative effects on other bones as well with increased incidents of fractures and bone cancers.

Arthritis and hip fractures are another long-term side effect.

Does our medical system consider fluoride when a patient presents with these conditions?

Some studies uncovered fluoride's negative effects on brain development.

Thankfully fluoride, when compared with many other insidious toxins, is easy to avoid.

We can just turn off the tap and avoid bottled water containing fluoride.

Please note that there are so many prescriptions which contain fluoride. Before taking any prescription, search to see if it contains this poison. Many of the psychopharmaceuticals are high on the list.

Dr. Paul Connett

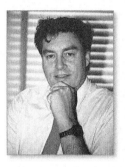

The most outspoken critic of fluoride use is Dr. Paul Connett, Professor Emeritus in Environmental Chemistry at St. Lawrence University in Canton, NY.

His B.A. is from Cambridge University in England with a Ph.D. in Chemistry from Dartmouth College in New Hampshire. He also co-authored *The Case Against Fluoride* in 2011.

Since 1985 he has given over 2,500 public presentations in 49 states, 7 provinces in Canada and 60 other countries.

One of his best talks can be found on YouTube. Search 'best fluoride documentary.'

Endocrine Disrupting Chemicals

Bisphenol A (BPA)

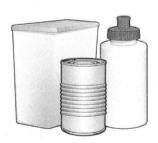

Let's begin with a group of toxins which are easy to cast out of our lives.

Many of these toxins are sanctioned by our governmental EPA telling or misleading us to believe they are relatively harmless and that the amounts we are exposed to are safe.

When we purchase plastic products containing endocrine disrupting chemicals, we are supporting corporate corruption. If we stop buying these plastic products and demand the use of safe alternatives, these companies will either change from consumer demands or fail.

We, the consumer, have the power and not lobbyists and EPA committees which are often influenced and officiated by corporations.

As you may know, BPA disrupts our endocrine function and all the organs and tissues which respond to hormones.

How to avoid BPA and other harmful plastics which are even BPA free?

Replace plastic containers with glass jars and stainless steel.

Avoid foods that come in cans unless the lining states BPA free.

Do not buy beverages in cans. Try switching to glass bottles.

Avoid handling glossy type paper receipts which contain BPA.

Avoid plastic utensils, plastic straws, plastic wraps like Saran Wrap, plastic cutting boards, plastic cups and plates, and no microwaving in plastic containers.

And what about our clothing?

We don't give much thought about what goes into making our synthetic, permanent press fabrics and clothing.

Ever ironed a polyester shirt with a little too much heat and noticed a strange smell?

Plastic garbage is shipped overseas and transformed into thread which is then used to make synthetic fabrics, furniture covering and carpets.

Buy all cotton apparel.

Dioxins

Dioxins are formed during many industrial processes when chlorine and bromine are burned in the presence of carbon and oxygen.

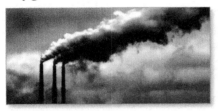

Dioxins disrupt male and female sex hormone signaling in the body. This is a bad thing!

Recent research has shown that exposure to low levels of dioxins in the womb and early in life can permanently affect sperm quality and sperm count in men during their prime reproductive years.

Dioxins are also very powerful carcinogens.

How to avoid them?

That's challenging since the ongoing industrial release of dioxins has widely contaminated the American food supply.

Products including meat, fish, milk, eggs and butter are most frequently contaminated.

Atrazine

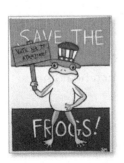

Researchers have found that exposure to even low levels of the herbicide atrazine can turn male frogs into females to produce completely viable eggs.

Atrazine is widely used on most corn crops in the United States and is consequently a pervasive contaminant in our drinking water.

Atrazine has been linked to breast tumors, delayed puberty, prostate inflammation in animals, and prostate cancer in men.

How to avoid it?

Buy organic produce and get a water filter certified to remove atrazine.

Phthalates

Old cells turn over or die as new cells surface. This is a normal regenerative process in the body.

But phthalates trigger what's known as "death-inducing signaling" or apoptosis causing our cells to die prematurely.

Studies have linked phthalates to hormonal changes, lower sperm count, less mobile sperm, birth defects, obesity, diabetes and thyroid irregularities.

How to avoid phthalates?

Avoid plastic food containers, children's toys (phthalates are already banned in some kid's products but not all) and plastic wrap made from PVC which has the recycling label #3.

Some personal care products also contain phthalates.

So, read the labels and avoid products that simply list 'added fragrance' since this catch-all term can mean hidden phthalates.

Perchlorate

Perchlorate is a component in rocket fuel and contaminates much of our produce and milk.

When perchlorate enters the body, it competes with the trace mineral iodide which thyroid cells require to make thyroid hormones.

This means that if perchlorate is occupying the channel or

symport through which iodide would be absorbed into a thyroid cell, you will slowly slip into hypothyroidism.

How to avoid it?

You can reduce perchlorate in your drinking water by installing a reverse osmosis filter or a water filtering system which guarantees perchlorate removal.

As for food, it's almost impossible to avoid perchlorate but you can reduce its harmful effects on the thyroid by taking an iodide, iodine and selenium supplement.

Perfluorinated Chemicals (PFCs)

Perfluorinated chemicals are used to make non-stick cookware.

These chemicals are so widespread and extraordinarily persistent that 99 percent of Americans have these chemicals in their bodies.

One type of PFC called PFOA has been linked to decreased sperm quality, low birth weight, kidney and thyroid disease, high cholesterol and other health issues.

How to avoid it?

Avoid non-stick pans as well as stain and water-resistant coatings on clothing, furniture and carpets.

Organophosphate Pesticides

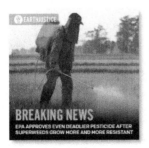

Neurotoxic organophosphate compounds were designed by the Nazis for chemical warfare during World War II.

After the war American scientists used the same chemistry to develop a long line of pesticides that target the nervous system of insects.

Despite many studies linking organophosphate exposure to negative effects on brain development, behavior and fertility, they are still among the more common pesticides in use today.

How to avoid it?

Buy organic produce.

Glycol Ethers

These chemicals are commonly found in solvents and paints, cleaning products, brake fluid and cosmetics.

The European Union says that some of these chemicals 'may damage fertility and the unborn child.'

Studies of painters have linked exposure to certain glycol ethers to blood abnormalities and lower sperm counts.

How to avoid it?

Avoid products with ingredients such as 2-butoxyethanol (EGBE) and methoxydiglycol (DEGME).

Toxins in the Home

I will try to keep this section simple even though there are thousands of household chemicals we can potentially be exposed to in our home.

First, it's very likely that every solution you use to clean sinks, countertops, ovens, refrigerators, bathtubs, shower stalls, clothes and glass are laden with chemicals.

Every chemical eventually finds its way into your body, especially if your home is kept closed and lacks circulation of outdoor air.

As you read through the following list please note that many of the harmful effects relate to acute, immediate exposure.

Long term exposures are subtle leading to chronic symptoms which may be difficult to track back to the use of these chemicals.

Antibacterial Cleaners

It may be safer to take your chances with the germs.

These cleaners contain triclosan, a form of dioxin, linked with weakened immune systems, decreased fertility, hormone disruption and birth defects.

There is also the danger of triclosan mixing with chlorinated tap water to form the deadly chlorinated dioxin.

Air Fresheners

Air fresheners stop you from smelling odors by coating nasal passages with an oily film or by releasing nerve deadening agents.

One of the most common ingredients is formaldehyde, a carcinogen, which may cause allergic reactions, dermatitis, headaches, mucous membrane irritations, joint and chest pain, depression, fatigue, dizziness and immune dysfunction.

Another main ingredient of air fresheners is phenol which can cause skin eruptions, cold sweats, convulsions, circulatory collapse and, in extreme cases, coma.

Dishwasher Detergents

These detergents are the number one cause of accidental child poisonings.

They contain a dry form of highly concentrated chlorine that is poisonous and has been known to produce skin irritations, burns, eye injuries and damage to other mucous membranes.

Residues that build up on dishes can also transfer into a hot meal.

At the end of the cycle, when you open your dishwasher, the odor you are inhaling is poisonous.

Oven Cleaners

Among the most dangerous household chemicals is sodium hydroxide, a derivative of lye.

It is so corrosive it can eat through the top layer of skin and cause severe tissue damage.

It's caustic to the eyes and lungs and can damage the nervous system.

These cleaners also contain benzene, toluene, xylene, methanol and ethyl benzene which are all known carcinogens.

Toxic fumes may also be released when the oven is set at the recommended temperature.

Carpet and Upholstery Shampoo

Designed to knock out stains, they may also take you out as well.

The main ingredient, perchloroethylene (the same chemical used in dry cleaning), is a known carcinogen and can damage the liver, kidneys and nervous system.

Another ingredient, ammonium hydroxide, is a corrosive which may cause irritation to eyes, skin and lungs.

Fumes from these cleaners are carcinogenic and may cause dizziness, sleepiness, nausea, loss of appetite and disorientation.

Toilet, Tub and Sink Cleaners

Highly toxic bathroom cleaners are a source of many

poisonings particularly since they are used in small, confined, often windowless spaces.

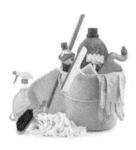

Most contain hydrochloric acid which irritates the skin, eyes and lungs and can potentially damage kidneys and liver.

They may also contain hypochlorite bleach, a corrosive, known to cause vomiting and pulmonary edema if inhaled.

These cleaners also contain benzene, toluene, xylene, methanol and ethyl benzene, which damage the nervous system and may cause birth defects.

Fragrances

All fragrances besides essential oils are made from petrochemicals.

Because these are aromatics, meaning they spread freely through the air, they are something to avoid.

Alternatives

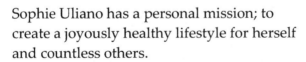

We can use some very basic ingredients to prepare many non-toxic multi-purpose cleansers for the kitchen and home.

Sophie Uliano has a personal mission; to create a joyously healthy lifestyle for herself and countless others.

She has a gift of speaking to the average woman struggling with an insanely busy and challenging life.

She was catapulted into natural products when she was horrifically burnt by a 'fireball' that exploded in her face while on a movie set in Canada. She was advised to go straight to a hospital burn unit which proposed skin grafts to restore 1st and 2nd degree burns to her face.

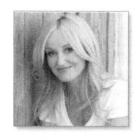

She insisted on the natural way and completely recovered using homeopathy, herbal preparations and creating a stress-free lifestyle. Within two weeks her skin was like new and never needed plastic surgery.

You can find numerous practical videos on how to prepare natural, chemical-free cleaning products by searching her name on YouTube.

One last thought.

If there's a warning on the label with advice to call the Center for Poison Control then remove the product from your home, especially if you have curious children.

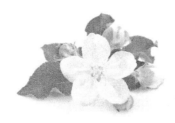

MOLDS IN THE HOME

I need to spend some time on the subject of mold because I've seen so many people with health issues related, in part, to either a present or previous exposure to mold.

Mold exposure can be one major underlying cause of illness and is seldom considered by our health professionals.

Common symptoms of mold exposure can relate to the lungs, sinuses, throat and skin but there can also be systemic physical effects leading to dysfunction of the immune system, liver, kidneys, pancreas and adrenals, as well as mental symptoms such as confusion, disorientation and brain fog.

Since the recovery of your health is dependent upon avoiding harmful influences, the identification of molds, especially in your home, is vital.

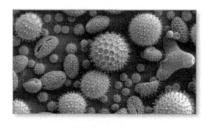

If molds are present in your home then your excretory organs may be too weak to effectively clear toxic residues released by your cells during purification, and you may become stuck in a healing crisis.

This is especially true for clients living in humid regions of the United States or in older homes with a history of water leaks and flooded basements.

Once molds are in the home they will never go away unless they are completely remediated.

This is a huge undertaking and, in more severely ill clients, even their furnishings and clothes must be discarded.

Some individuals are more sensitive or susceptible to molds, meaning their immune system has become so compromised that mycotoxins penetrate past the body's protective barriers.

Susceptibility

I've noticed that people with a history of excessive use of antibiotics are particularly susceptible to mycotoxins.

I suspect that a person is being exposed to molds when some of the following symptoms are present.

- Sensitive to fragrances and perfumes (this can also point to a molybdenum deficiency)
- Alcohol intolerance
- Recurring vaginal infections
- Recurring urinary tract infections
- Chronic sinus issues
- Recurring lung issues
- Cravings for sweets and fruit
- Itching or rashes in folds of skin
- Athlete's foot
- Recurring sore throats
- Chronic allergies
- Waking tired even after a full night's sleep

Of course, all people with mold issues have fatigue and foggy brains yet these symptoms do not automatically point to a mold issue.

So, if you suspect mold and mycotoxin exposure what's the best approach to take?

Mold Remediation

First of all, stop filling the bowl.

Do a thorough search of your home from top to bottom. If you find mold growth in your home tape a plastic barrier around it and seek professional help.

If you find molds in your basement be sure the spores are not entering the rest of your home through your duct system.

If air circulates from the basement into the rest of your home tape cardboard over the vent to prevent basement air from entering the rest of your home.

If there's not a door between your living quarters and the basement then put up a plastic barrier.

If you suspect mold (musty smell) but don't see it, use mold test plates to check various rooms. You can buy these on the immunolytics.com site.

What about getting a professional to check your home for mold?

Here's a story about a woman with health issues primarily from mold exposure.

Under the dark field microscope, we could see mold in her blood, and she had many of the characteristic symptoms of mold exposure.

Before we started any IV therapies, I wanted her to be sure their home was free of mold, otherwise she would not recover her health.

Her family sought a mold remediation expert to examine and test their home.

Their home got a clean bill of health.

Therefore, she had a three Zotzmann ozone treatments alternating with intravenous vitamin C.

Checking her blood again under the microscope, her blood was clear of mold and she was feeling much better.

About a month later she returned with a recurrence of her symptoms and the mold was showing up again under the microscope.

Even though the expert claimed her home was free of mold I knew it wasn't because of this recurrence.

The mother searched for an alternative way to examine their home and found molddogs.com.

It just so happened that the 'mold' dog sniffed out nine spots around their home and when the walls were torn down, mold growth was visibly obvious.

Ozone to Kill Molds

If mold growth is minor, then consider purchasing a high output ozone generator. A generator on Amazon is not that expensive and you'll want to run it periodically.

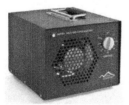 You should not breathe ozone, so close doors when ozonating each room and run towels across the space between the door and floor since ozone is heavier than air.

Open all cabinets and closet doors in rooms and, depending upon the generator's output, run it for 6-10 hours.

Remember that when you run this generator, air from this room should not circulate into the rest of the house if you are home.

It's also wise to clear molds from your duct system by placing the generator next to one of the air intake vents and leaving the thermostat fan button in the 'on' position. This will circulate ozone throughout all the ducts and your entire home. You should not be in your home during this time.

Upon returning to your home turn off the generator, open all the windows and remain outside for a while.

One cause of mold is high humidity even though molds do grow in dryer climates. When windows are shut and very little outside air is circulating through your home, humidity levels will rise.

This humidity encourages mold growth.

Purification Therapies for Mold Symptoms

The next step then is to empty the bowl.

Regular saunas are very important. Do as many cycles of hot sauna/cold showers as you can but you should not feel tired after.

Saunas help to remove some of the mycotoxin residues stored in the sub-dermal fat layer.

Intravenous vitamin C and other nutrients such as glutathione support your body's ability to recover and can really help to turn your symptoms around.

The two primary reasons for the vitamin C IV are to increase the activity of white blood cells and to support your adrenals which are likely exhausted from living in a moldy environment and the chronic systemic mold.

Some supplements and homeopathies are also helpful.

The IV therapies which are essential for decreasing systemic mold in the body are the ozone Zotzmann treatments and the UBI.

I no longer use expensive lab testing for mold.

I have found the viewing of a small finger prick of blood under a dark-field microscope to be the most reliable way to assess mold issues and a simple, inexpensive way to evaluate a person's progress during therapies.

Candida & Mold

I mentioned the relationship between mold and the overuse of antibiotics.

Very often I've found that most people with mold issues have an overgrowth of Candida in the gut with the symptoms of mold and Candida being similar.

Therefore, besides the steps mentioned regarding mold, a person must also improve their gut health by dealing with the Candida.

This requires a dietary regiment to avoid foods that feed Candida, to take a high-quality probiotic and to use anti-candida supplements.

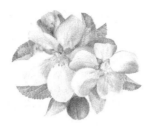

FSM Frequencies

Here we present the various Frequency Specific Microcurrents (FSM) which are effective in reducing pain and inflammatory cytokines and improving Central Nervous System glandular functions.

Some physical and mental symptoms originate in the brain as a result of head and spine traumas, chronic infections and inflammation, the use of synthetic drugs, and as a result of the three primary causes already covered.

Treating the glands of the brain, to bring them back into balance and optimal function, is extremely challenging, but the application of micro frequencies can correct and balance these difficult to reach organs.

I have often referred to the need for increasing the ATP production of mitochondria, and FSM has been proven to stimulate this beneficial effect.

Before covering these frequencies, it is interesting to know the historical use of frequencies over the last 100 years, and why the use of microcurrents will bring about a new and revolutionary approach to treating a wide range of conditions.

I have spent the last few decades helping patients to manage their symptoms, addressing their downstream symptoms, but not until we applied microcurrents did we witness profound improvements.

This is because we can now affect deep tissues, glands and organs with healing, regenerative frequencies.

FSM History

In medicine we have become overly reliant and dependent upon synthetic chemicals.

The breadth of medical practice used to be much broader, encompassing a wide variety of approaches which, these days, would be included in alternative medicine.

In the late 1800s there was a great interest in using electromagnetism for healing.

Thousands of medical and osteopathic physicians were drawn to electric therapies for treating their patients.

One physician was Dr. Albert Abrams, MD, who practiced in San Francisco, California, from 1914 until 1937. He founded a society and a publication as the means for physicians to share and communicate their research and treatments. Many, many

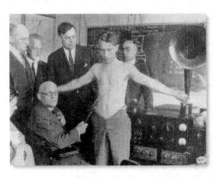

physicians would visit Abrams to learn more about the use of electric current treatments.

In 1934 the American Medical Association mandated that drugs and surgery were the only accepted tools of medicine, and that any physician using electromagnetic therapies would lose their license.

116

These physicians and their devices went into hiding.

Dr. Harry Van Gelder, an osteopath and naturopath, bought a practice in Vancouver, British Columbia, that came with one of these early electromedical machines, along with a list of frequencies specific for certain conditions.

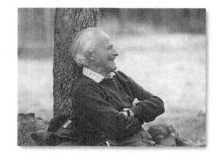

Eventually he moved to Ojai, California, with patients coming from across the United States and Canada.

A student of Chiropractic, George Douglas, heard about Dr. Gelder's work and, in 1980, spent three months working with Gelder to learn his methods.

Dr. Carolyn McMakin, DC, was a student of Douglas', who incorporated micro frequencies into her practice, and is now the most knowledgeable and experienced FSM practitioner.

She has written two books and devotes the majority of her time to FSM seminars for licensed physicians in North America, Europe and other continents.

What Is Frequency Specific Microcurrent Therapy?

Explaining how FSM works is challenging.

We must step outside the box of what we know in medicine, into the realm of physics, especially quantum physics, that matter has characteristics of both particles and waves, simultaneously.

This leads us back to Einstein, who envisioned an electromagnetic wave, such as light, being also a particle, later called a photon.

Every tissue in your body is composed of cells, and every cell is made of atoms (electrons, protons, neutrons, photons and others), and every atom is made of subatomic particles which fluctuate between matter and energy packets.

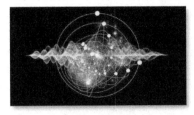

There is little doubt, in the world of quantum physics, that we are both matter and energy.

From this point of view, we are not necessarily held together by elastic connective tissue and fascia, but bonds of invisible energy and frequencies.

The frequencies emitted by a liver cell are different from the frequencies emitted by a heart cell.

I know this is a stretch beyond what we are familiar with, because we have resided our entire life within this solid body.

But sometimes, when you are still, when all the surrounding chatter and clutter of life has quieted, you can, if you get in touch with your body, feel the sensations of energy within you.

I like to think of it as a symphony, that all the parts of me, the varied instruments (tissues and glands) are sounding their tune (frequencies) and their harmony is felt as a singular, perceptible vibration.

You cannot hear this symphony, but you can feel it.

Each part of us has a resonance, a subtle frequency, which emits a tiny current of energy.

And this energy can fluctuate depending upon the health and vitality of the tissue.

What if there's a way to restore vitality to a tissue, to increase its frequency, to move it in the direction of health?

I understand this explanation falls far short of explaining the miraculous energy within each of us, and how FSM therapy is working at this depth of restoration.

On one level, how it works may not be possible to fully explain, but I have witnessed the benefits.

Story

A man came to us with burning pain and numbness on the left side of his body along with frequent urination, both of which he'd had for the last 10 years.

He had visited so many physicians to the point of complete frustration and depression.

After two FSM treatments one week apart, his symptoms were 90% better, with his last treatment being a month ago.

With this kind of result, as well as many other examples, who cares how it works.

It may not matter to think quantum particles and waves (frequencies).

It has provided a way to treat deep internal structures such as the brain.

This means the primary underlying issue with Fibromyalgia, Central Nervous System dysregulation, can be addressed.

Pairing Frequencies

The FSM unit has two frequency output channels which run simultaneously.

One channel, channel A, emits microcurrent frequencies corresponding to the 'condition' of a tissue.

These could include the following but there are many others;

- Inflammation
- Adhesions (scars)

- Swelling or edema
- Toxins of which there are many
- Infections of which there are many
- Hardening or induration
- Trauma

The other channel, channel B, emits microcurrent frequencies related to 'specific' tissues.

One pair of frequencies (channels A and B) could address 'inflammation' of the 'nerves.'

Another pair increases the ATP production of mitochondria.

Another pair decreases inflammatory cytokines.

These are all possible with FSM, and I know of no other way to do this in such a simple, elegant and rapid way.

I hope I have conveyed the usefulness of FSM.

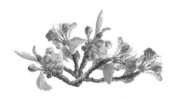

The Psychology of Health

You could say, everything that happens to us in our life is meant to be, that we might even unconsciously ask for events or experiences which help us to grow and to evolve, to become more of the person we deeply desire to become.

Is is our fate or more likely our soul guiding us towards the deeper reasons for our brief earthly existence?

Here I relate a personal story as an example.

When I was 8 years of age I had an experience which helped shape who I am today.

It was a blistering hot afternoon and I was playing baseball in the backyard with friends.

The closest source of cool water was in the laundry room just off the backdoor of our home.

I normally had to climb on top of the dryer and bend over the sink to drink from the tap.

This day I saw a metal watering can on the concrete floor below the sink, and I drank deeply.

Within seconds I started convulsing and vomiting.

The next thing I remember was lying on the floor of the

passenger's side of our car and the howling of the horn as my mother raced to the nearest hospital a half hour away.

I fell unconscious.

Apparently my stomach was pumped and I was rushed to a hospital in San Francisco.

I remained in a coma for two weeks.

My only recollection during this time was this sense of leaving my body and floating in a heavy atmosphere of bliss.

I had never experienced this before in my life.

It was heavenly.

Then I approached this luminous being and since I was raised a Catholic I thought, damn, this must be God.

We did not exchange words but I felt welcomed and unconditionally loved. This sense permeated my entire being.

After a while of basking in this radiance I was offered two choices.

I could remain where I was or return to my earthly existence.

My 1st instinct was to remain since how I felt in these surroundings was delicious.

But then I remembered my mother and how much she loved me and I her, yet, in some ways, how unhappy she was in her marriage.

I felt, 'I want to return to help her,' and in that instant, like a dream, I awoke.

The hospital room was pristine white and the shear white curtains billowed through the room like clouds, from the San Francisco bay breeze.

There was my mother sitting by the side of my bed.

I think I must have had amnesia about this experience because I really didn't recollect it until years later.

Experiences like this always seem to leave a core message deep within.

For me it was, 'to help.'

I relay this story as it relates to the psychology of health, our attitudes around suffering and how ill-health provides us with opportunities.

If we are ill we can respond in may different ways;

- Why me?
- Poor me.
- Doc, just give me a pill.
- I want to learn more about why I am not well.
- What is the lesson I am meant to learn?
- What am I doing that has created this condition?
- What am I not doing that has created this condition?
- What changes do I need to make in my life to correct this condition?

So how do we move from complaining to being curious and constructive, to somehow develop gratitude for becoming ill as if it is a blessing in disguise so we may live more consciously and to navigate our life towards our True North Star?

In this light, we possess many spiritual capacities which we are unaware of, which can be further developed through practice.

Developing Trust

During my second year at the National University of Natural Medicine, six of us made a pact to go through a week long water fast.

We met each day to talk about our experiences.

Some of us experienced slight headaches, nausea and occassional aches and pains but overall we all had greater mental clarity and energy.

We all accepted these minor discomforts because we knew they were part of the detoxification process and this acceptance or positive attitude was extremely important.

During purification there needs to be this sense of surrendering and allowing the wisdom within us to take over and to do what it does best, which is to bring us back into balance and to reestablish our health.

This surrendering is facilitated by relaxation and turning inward, a kind of meditative state. This relaxed state of trust will help the wisdom within you to reestablish homeostasis more rapidly.

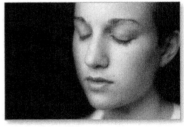

With the symptoms that arise during purification we don't want to counteract or suppress them.

We do not resist.

We just watch and observe them with a positive attitude.

They will pass.

Of course during this time we can support this wisdom with purification therapies.

Stepping into a purification program requires the following

mindset.

- Believe in the wisdom and intelligence of your innate physician.

- Know that at some point symptoms will arise when impurities are flushed from cells.

- Shift your attitude about symptoms and learn to surrender during the healing crisis.

I want to clarify one more thing about symptoms.

I know this may sound strange but as the body becomes stronger it allows toxins to be released from cells, like peeling back the layers of an onion.

The strange thing is that the first toxins released by the body are the ones we were most recently exposed to and then, working down through a chronological history, the oldest toxins will be excreted last.

Now I have been referring primarily to physical symptoms but psychological symptoms will arise as well.

And somehow we have toxins associated with emotions or reminders of past events.

As a toxic layer is released we may experience an associated memory or emotion.

As toxins are being released we can drift into a multitude of emotions and thoughts.

How can we develop an attitude of surrendering when it comes to these mental and emotional symptoms?

It's pretty easy to simply observe pain or nausea.

It is definitely more challenging to observe a thought or emotion such as sadness because they seem to be so real.

Yet each of us has an inborn capacity to observe, which means we can simply watch our thoughts and emotions without engaging in them.

This capacity allows us to remain detached and therefore less likely to believe them.

After all, what we are experiencing during sadness is often simply the biochemistry of hormones as they float through our blood stream.

Your Faculty of Observation

Just to add some clarity, besides your innate physician you also possess a faculty I refer to as our 'Observer.'

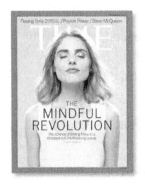

This capacity helps you to live life with greater awareness and is sometimes referred to as 'Mindfulness.'

Your Observer watches the physical sensations of your body.

It watches your thoughts and feelings as they rise and fall.

It is separate from your physical body, separate from your emotions and separate from your thoughts.

Your Observer does not 'do' anything.

It simply watches, and no matter what it witnesses it remains neutral, calm, non-judgemental and somewhat curious.

This faculty is often developed through the practice of meditation when we sit, watch and enter a space of neutrality and serenity.

Yet it is a practice which must become a way of life.

What I spoke of before, about surrendering to our symptoms during purification and allowing our innate physician to do what it does best, applies here.

We do not resist what comes to the forefront of our awareness because what we resist will persist.

The psychology of health means;

- Trusting this miraculous wisdom within
- Letting go and surrendering to this wisdom
- Physically sensing this wisdom as it courses througout the entire body, as it gently but surely brings you back to health. Your attention accelerates its activity.
- Learning to listen to this wisdom
- Developing our capacity to simply witness
- Developing gratitude for what our condition is teaching us and the direction it is guiding us.

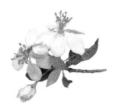

LAB TESTING & BIOCHEMISTRY

Sometimes with a chronic condition, various glands begin to falter, and their respective hormones begin to deviate from normal.

This will negatively affect every cell of the body and brain and produce both physical and mental symptoms.

It is therefore important to evaluate each person to see to what extent their biochemistry is slipping away from optimal.

Seldom have we seen just one dysfunctional gland or organ but rather more of a cascading effect where several glands are struggling.

We have found that even when we address the three primary causes of symptoms, if we fail to support and correct biochemical and hormonal imbalances then the rapidity of a person's recovery is unduly and unnecessarily hindered.

The most common imbalances we find correspond to the pancreas, thyroid, adrenals and reproductive organs.

Here are the most common issues we find, the types of labs

which help to assess deficiencies or imbalances and how to hopefully correct them.

Blood Sugar Dysregulation

The two most common issues people have around blood sugar are when it's too high or too low.

You would think that a simple blood glucose test, when having not eaten for 12 hours prior (fasting), would be enough to determine issues, but for many people their greatest challenge is just before eating and during the two hours after.

Some people know when they slip into low blood sugar (hypoglycemia) because they experience weakness, various moods and sometimes dizziness, but these are not always the case.

For about 10 years we ran sophisticated testing of blood, urine and saliva. One part of this testing included a single fasting blood glucose and then frequent glucose testing for three hours after a sugar drink.

I was surprised to hear people say about an hour after the sweet drink, 'Doc, I'm sinking. I need something to eat. My blood sugar is plummeting.'

So we'd check their blood sugar and found it was actually high.

Yes, their cells were starved for glucose, but it was a metabolic issue; their cells were not absorbing glucose.

So how can we know if there's a blood sugar dysfunction without going through the torture of a glucose tolerance test?

The lab test Hemoglobin A1c (HA1c for short) tells us a person's average blood sugar over the past three months.

So, let's say a person has a perfect fasting glucose of 85.

Then we check their HA1c which calculates out to 85 as well.

Most docs would say this result is great because they are looking for a high HA1c which points to diabetes.

But what might this HA1c of 85 really tell us?

After a meal the glucose in our blood rises to let's say 130. Then insulin enters our blood and shuttles glucose out of our blood and into our cells.

Now our blood glucose is falling.

How far down it drops will depend upon several hormonal factors.

If it drops down to 60 then we are in hypoglycemia and we may experience various unpleasant symptoms.

Remember that the HA1c blood test indicates an average of the peaks and valleys of our blood sugar over 90 days.

So, if the peaks are around 130 and the valleys are around 60 our average blood sugar will be around 85.

This means that a person with a fasting blood sugar of 85 and a calculated HA1c of 85 has been falling into hypoglycemia throughout the day.

If another person's HA1c calculates out to say 140, they are prediabetic because their blood sugar after a meal goes up and stays there for too long.

There are many ideas about why this happens.

- Too little insulin produced. Glucose is not being shuttled out of the blood into cells.

- Insulin insensitivity; plenty of insulin but the gates in cell membranes are not opening to allow glucose in.

- Too many fat cells.

131

- Trace mineral deficiencies such as chromium.

With these results, comparing fasting glucose to the HA1c, specific dietary modifications can be made.

Low blood sugar can also relate to adrenal fatigue.

The adrenals make the hormone cortisol which plays many important secondary roles in the body.

One role is to signal fat cells to liberate free fatty acids which are fuel for cells.

Normally when our blood glucose is dropping during the day or night the body senses this decline and sounds the message, 'Feed me!'

Some people are too busy to listen to this hunger signal or maybe they have decided to lose weight by skipping a meal.

Some people have digestive issues and feel better if they don't eat.

But if the blood sugar continues to drop, the 'fight or flight' alarm goes off, calling the adrenals to make cortisol.

Uh oh! Adrenal fatigue means there's too little cortisol and the blood sugar continues to drop.

Battle stations!! 'Adrenals, release another hormone!'

And adrenaline comes to the rescue.

Adrenaline may save the day by averting a coma but there are many harmful side effects of too much adrenaline including inflammation.

Adrenal Hormones

There are several indications or symptoms of adrenal fatigue which equate to low cortisol production.

- Hypoglycemia as you just read.

- Dizziness usually when rising from sitting to standing.

- Eyes sensitive to light

- Lack of appetite

- Insomnia

- A desire for salt

But remember that adrenal fatigue always has causes.

- Low thyroid hormones

- Chronic infections

- Infected root canals

- All toxic burdens

- Low fat diets

- Chronic stress

- Insomnia

The most accurate way to check cortisol levels is through saliva hormone testing.

All hormones in the blood are either attached to a protein carrier, like being on a bus, or detached from the protein carrier and referred to as free.

These free hormones are small enough to leave the blood stream, pass through the lymph fluid to then enter cells. This lymph, which has the free hormones, is saliva.

Saliva hormone testing is an accurate way of checking the free forms of hormones.

This way, by collecting four saliva samples throughout the day from the morning until before bed, we can have an accurate assessment of cortisol levels.

How high or how low cortisol levels are gives us an idea about how to address an underlying cortisol issue.

Controlling blood sugar, meaning to prevent hypoglycemia, is a crucial step in helping with adrenal fatigue.

There are many other solutions to correct adrenal fatigue but, as you will see, there are other reasons for fatigue that may not be related to the adrenals.

Thyroid Hormones

You likely know most of the symptoms of low thyroid hormones.

We can do a thyroid blood panel which tells us about thyroid hormones in the blood, but it doesn't tell us whether they are getting into cells and binding to their respective receptors within the cells.

Even when a person has optimal blood levels of thyroid hormones, if they have dysfunctional mitochondria, they will still experience low thyroid hormone symptoms.

But lab testing is a place to start.

Knowing which thyroid hormones to test to get a comprehensive overview is extremely important.

I will describe each thyroid hormone, their interactions and what their function is.

TSH (thyroid stimulating hormone) is produced by the pituitary gland in the brain.

This gland is always monitoring levels of thyroid hormones in the blood.

If thyroid hormones in the blood start to decline, then the pituitary will secrete more TSH.

This hormone travels through the blood and binds to its respective receptor on the membrane of a thyroid cell telling it to make more thyroid hormones.

The secretion of thyroid hormones from a thyroid cell then enter the blood steam, and when the pituitary senses this increase it will then slow down its production and secretion of TSH.

Ideally this is how it's supposed to work; thyroid hormones go down, TSH goes up… thyroid hormones go up, TSH goes down.

When triggered by TSH, thyroid cells secrete primarily the thyroid hormone called T4 or Thyroxine with the number 4 representing 4 atoms of iodine on this hormone.

T4 is the most abundant thyroid hormone produced by thyroid cells, but it is not the primary thyroid hormone which activates the function of all our cells.

There's an enzyme in the body which removes one atom of iodine from the T4 to make T3 (3 atoms of iodine) and this T3 is a lot more potent or stimulating compared with the T4.

Now remember, all hormones in the blood are either attached to a protein carrier or they are detached and referred to as free.

So, we have the blood test for Thyroxine T4, also referred to as the Total T4, which tells us the T4 bound to its protein carrier and the T4 that is detached, or free.

We want to know the Total T4 and we want to know the Free T4 because it's the Free T4 which is small enough to leave the blood stream.

So thus far I have covered three of the thyroid hormones that need to be checked through lab testing; TSH, T4 (Total) and Free T4.

Then we need to know the levels of Free T3 since this is the most activating thyroid hormone.

Very little T3 is secreted by thyroid cells.

Remember there's an enzyme that pulls one atom of iodine off the T4 to make T3.

Sometimes this enzyme is not working well which slows this conversion of Free T4 to Free T3.

Low Free T3 will cause low thyroid hormone symptoms.

You can have optimal levels of Free T4 but low levels of Free T3 and therefor experience low thyroid hormone symptoms.

So it is very important to include Free T3 along with the other hormones already mentioned.

Now let's look at a lab's reference range which all physicians use to know whether a lab result is 'normal.'

Every lab result is given a reference range and is found on every lab report.

How is this reference range determined?

Take 1,000 people and draw their blood to check, let's say, T4.

They gather all the 1,000 results, clip 15% off the high results and 15% off the low results, and now you have the reference range.

So, if your result falls within this range, even if it is at the very bottom of the range, you will be told it's normal.

But we don't want normal, we want optimal.

Let's backtrack for a moment.

Say you have all the signs and symptoms of hypothyroidism.

You go to your doctor and he or she says they'll check your thyroid.

One doc may only check TSH and the result falls within the reference range.

'Your thyroid is normal and not a problem,' you hear the physician say.

Now you know better because this single test does not tell you if your thyroid cells are even responding to the TSH.

Another doc will check both TSH and Free T4.

At least now we'll know how well your thyroid cells are responding to TSH.

But very often a person's Free T4 will fall within the lower part of the reference range and again the result is normal, but it's actually suboptimal and will be a partial cause of low thyroid symptoms.

And with checking the TSH and the Free T4 we still don't know how well the body is converting the Free T4 to Free T3, which again is the most important thyroid hormone to check.

Why don't docs check the Free T3?

Because they don't know how to interpret the result and what to do about it.

They don't know the cause of poor conversion from Free T4 to Free T3.

Most don't know how to prescribe T3 medication even though it is a prescription.

And why don't they normally check for a thyroid autoimmune condition called Hashimoto's?

Because they don't understand the causes of this condition (thyroid inflammation) or how to treat it.

Just one final word so you can grasp this situation.

There are two types of hypothyroidism.

On labs, both types show low thyroid hormones (T4, Free T4 and Free T3).

The first type, called primary hypothyroidism, is when TSH is high.

The pituitary is sensing low thyroid hormones in the blood and is secreting a lot of TSH to stimulate thyroid cells to make more thyroid hormones.

But the thyroid cells are unable to produce enough thyroid hormones, so thyroid hormones remain low and TSH remains high.

There are several reasons for this.

One reason is thyroid cells don't have the nutrients required to assemble the thyroid hormones.

We are back to the first primary cause of chronic illness, nutrient deficiencies.

These nutrients are <u>iodide</u>, selenium, zinc and iron.

If any of these are lacking, then the assembly line for making thyroid hormones slows down.

Besides these nutrient deficiencies, you must also consider mitochondrial dysfunction, and the importance of providing nutrients they require.

So, this covers the first type of hypothyroidism (primary hypothyroidism): Increased TSH and low thyroid hormones.

The other type is called secondary hypothyroidism.

Remember both types have low thyroid hormone levels in the blood, and both suffer from symptoms of hypothyroidism.

With secondary hypothyroidism, TSH is low.

This means that the pituitary is not working well and is unable to secrete enough TSH to signal thyroid cells to make thyroid hormones.

Reasons for low TSH when thyroid hormones are low are

numerous and I won't get into them.

Most of the time what I've seen is that older people are more likely to have secondary hypothyroidism.

So, you can see now how ridiculous it is for a doctor to check only TSH as the single marker for determining if a person has thyroid issues.

I do believe there is a place for prescribing thyroid hormones and can be important when addressing the three primary causes of chronic illness, especially the first (nutritional deficiencies) since thyroid hormones are required for digestion and assimilation of nutrients.

Cholesterol

One of the most important nutrients is cholesterol.

It is needed for healthy cellular membranes including the nervous system and brain.

Cholesterol is also required for making all our steroid hormones.

Steroid hormones include all the female and male hormones and those made by the adrenals.

And just because your blood cholesterol may be high, I suspect that it's the fresh cholesterol taken with each meal throughout the day that's important.

Here's a brief story.

A 38-year-old woman contacted me for an appointment. She lived in Texas and had all the typical hypothyroid symptoms as well as several others.

She had already had her thyroid hormones checked which showed suboptimal thyroid hormone levels.

I put her on a thyroid prescription.

139

After a month she didn't feel much improvement, so I asked her to approach her physician with a list of labs I recommended.

I suspected blood sugar issues and adrenal fatigue.

About two weeks later she called me in tears.

Her cholesterol was 365 with normal being less than 199.

I confirmed that she had been fasting for 12 hours before the blood draw.

She was scared because her doctor told her she would die of a heart attack in five years if she didn't control her cholesterol by taking a lipid lowering drug.

She was also frustrated because she had been on a low-fat diet to lose weight which hadn't helped much.

She was also frightened because of a family history of elevated cholesterol.

I tried to calm her, telling her I didn't believe that in most cases there was any relationship between eating cholesterol foods and elevated fasting cholesterol.

I asked her if she'd like to try an experiment for five weeks.

She agreed because she didn't want to take a prescription to lower her cholesterol.

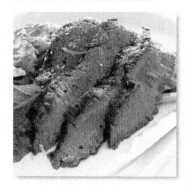

I asked the question, if she went out to a restaurant to celebrate her birthday and didn't think about gaining weight or her elevated cholesterol, what would she order.

Immediately she said a slice of prime rib.

I told her I wanted her to eat beef once a day and even twice daily if possible.

'Dr. Haskell, are you sure? What if…I die?'

I told her it would only be for five weeks and nothing was going to happen.

She hesitated but we had developed a good relationship, enough for her to trust me.

OK, she agreed and planned to follow my advice and to have another fasting lab test for cholesterol in five weeks.

I crossed my fingers.

She called in five weeks and I could immediately tell by her voice that she was happy.

Phew!

I had been a little apprehensive about the call.

'Dr. Haskell, my cholesterol is down to 198 and I feel great. Almost all my symptoms are 90% better.'

She had lost about 30 pounds.

I relate this story in part to show how important cholesterol rich foods are for blood sugar regulation and improving adrenal function.

I believe her low production of cortisol due to her low-fat diet was why her cells were unable to utilize the thyroid hormone prescription.

SUMMARY & HIGHLIGHTS

I hope this information has provided you with a fresh perspective on ways you can recover your health.

Here are some highlights around what's been covered.

- Nature, especially the nature within you, is the source of healing.

- You possess a miraculous innate physician which is dedicated to helping you to recover your health.

- Secure a mental attitude of respect and appreciation for this wisdom.

- This wisdom speaks to you through physical and mental symptoms, your conscience, intuition, instincts and common sense.

- It is your responsibility to support this wisdom and to learn its language.

- Most conditions are due to nutritional deficiencies, harmful environmental toxins and pathogens.

- These three causes penetrate deep into the cell leading to mitochondrial dysfunction.

- Stop filling the bowl.

- Investigate and eradicate toxins in your home and your food.

- Empty the bowl.

- Use purification therapies to excrete toxins from the cells and body; saunas, colon hydrotherapy, lymphatic drainage and IV therapies.

- Use intravenous therapies to improve nutrient levels, to support the immune system, to reduce pathogens and environmental toxins, and to improve the pathways of detoxification.

- Ensure optimal nutrient levels using fresh organic low-glycemic juices.

- Clean up the gut and restore the population of beneficial bacteria.

- Realize that the vitality deep within your body and soul can never be restored through artificial means.

- Invest in your health otherwise your savings and income will be consumed by medical expenses.

I ask you one final question.

Will there ever be a magic pill that can restore the health of anyone with a chronic condition?

If there is, I would certainly not hesitate for a moment to prescribe it.

What physician would not do the same, wanting to relieve the suffering of their patient?

But as you now know, not only is our existence a miracle, it is beyond mysterious, far beyond the intelligence of man to even conceive of God's miraculous creation.

But if we can at least remember that another human is a

miraculous creation, then maybe we can also fathom how we can help a person to lift themselves out of the darkness of blind ignorance, confusion and naivete.

Made in the USA
Middletown, DE
06 April 2022

63669800R00089